D0226973

High Density Lipoprotein Cholesterol: The New Target

A Handbook for Clinicians

Third Edition

Professor Philip Barter
Director
The Heart Research Institute
Sydney, Australia

Professor Kerry-Anne Rye
Head, Lipid Research Group
The Heart Research Institute
Sydney, Australia

Published by Sherborne Gibbs Limited

3 Duchess Place, Edgbaston, Birmingham

ISBN: 978-1-905036-10-3

Printed in the United Kingdom by
Caric Print Limited, Bournemouth, Dorset
in association with Stephens & George Magazines Limited.

Design and Production: Michel le Sueur Corporate Design
Layout, Illustration Rendering and Typesetting: Jonathan Berndt.

Contents

4S - Scandinavian Simvastatin Survival Study

LIPID - Long-Term Intervention with Pravastatin in Ischaemic Disease study

CARE - Cholesterol And Recurrent Events trial

HPS - Heart Protection Study

WOSCOPS - West Of Scotland Coronary Prevention Study

AFCAPS/TexCAPS - Air Force/Texas Coronary Atherosclerosis Prevention Study

ASCOT - Anglo-Scandinavian Cardiac Outcomes Trial

CARDS - Collaborative AtoRvastatin in Diabetes Study

A direct involvement of plasma cholesterol in the development and progression of atherosclerotic cardiovascular risk is one of the best-proven cases in modern medicine. A strong, positive relationship between the concentration of low density lipoprotein cholesterol (LDL-C) and the future risk of cardiovascular events has been observed in many large-scale population studies and the benefits of reducing LDL-C levels has been proven beyond doubt in intervention studies.

Trial Name	Trial Type	Drug Used	Reduction in CHD Events (%)
4S	Secondary prevention in subjects with high LDL-C	Simvastatin	34
LIPID	Secondary prevention in subjects with average LDL-C	Pravastatin	24
CARE	Secondary prevention in subjects with average LDL-C	Pravastatin	24
HPS	Primary and secondary prevention in high risk subjects	Simvastatin	25
WOSCOPS	Primary prevention in subjects with high LDL-C	Pravastatin	31
AFCAPS/ TexCAPS	Primary prevention in subjects with low LDL-C	Lovastatin	25
ASCOT	Primary prevention in hypertension	Atorvastatin	36
CARDS	Primary prevention in type 2 diabetes	Atorvastatin	37

Table I.1. CHD event reduction in intervention trials with statins

Yet, despite the impressive cardioprotective effects of aggressive LDL-C lowering, it is becoming apparent that LDL-C reduction alone may have begun to reach the point of diminishing returns. It is also apparent that, despite highly effective lowering of LDL-C, the residual risk in many people remains unacceptably high. Much of this residual risk relates to the presence of a low level of high density lipoprotein cholesterol (HDL-C).

It has been known for many years that the concentration of HDL-C correlates inversely with cardiovascular risk. For example, the Framingham Heart Study showed that people whose HDL-C level was less than 35 mg/dL (0.91 mmol/L) at the beginning of the study had a future coronary risk more than eight times that in subjects whose HDL-C level was greater than 65 mg/dL (1.68 mmol/L). In the Prospective Cardiovascular Münster (PROCAM) Study, men with HDL-C levels less than 35 mg/dL (0.91 mmol/L) at baseline had a six-year coronary risk about four times that in men whose HDL-C was greater than 35 mg/dL (0.91 mmol/L). In each case, the excess risk associated with lower HDL-C levels was independent of LDL-C level observed in those with high, average or low concentrations of LDL-C.

These, and other population studies, strongly support the view that raising the level of HDL-C should be considered as a therapeutic target of importance comparable to that of lowering LDL-C. Despite this, HDL-C raising remains a secondary goal in most guidelines, including the recently amended National Cholesterol Education Program (NCEP) guidelines. In part, this reflects the paucity of therapeutic options available for raising HDL-C.

Thus, cholesterol-related cardiovascular risk should be attacked on two fronts: the negative aspects of plasma cholesterol should be attacked by reducing the level of LDL-C, while the positive aspects should be boosted by raising the level of HDL-C. This concept has been further strengthened by the results of the INTERHEART Study in which the ratio of apoB to apoA-I (reflecting the ratio of LDL to HDL) was of enormous power in predicting future myocardial infarction in a large cohort of subjects of widely differing ethnic origin.

The importance of targeting HDLs as a therapeutic strategy is further highlighted by the fact that there is an alarming and escalating worldwide epidemic of low HDL states such as type 2 diabetes and the metabolic syndrome.

The time of HDLs as a therapeutic target has arrived.

It is now necessary for physicians to understand what HDLs are and to know when and how to act to enhance the protection provided by these lipoproteins.

So, what are HDLs? Where are they formed? How are they regulated? What is their function? How do they protect against atherosclerosis? Why is the plasma level of HDL-C low in some people and how can it be raised? These and many other questions are addressed in this book.

References

LaRosa JC. Reduction of serum LDL-C levels: a relationship to clinical benefits. *Am J Cardiovasc Drugs* 2003;**3**:271-81.

Expert Panel on Detection, Evaluation, and Treatment of High Blood Cholesterol in Adults. Executive Summary of the Third Report of the National Cholesterol Education Program (NCEP) Expert Panel on Detection, Evaluation, and Treatment of High Blood Cholesterol in Adults (Adult Treatment Panel III). *JAMA* 2001;**285**:2486-97.

Grundy SM, Cleeman JI, Merz CN, Brewer HB Jr, Clark LT, Hunninghake DB, Pasternak RC, Smith SC Jr, Stone NJ; National Heart, Lung, and Blood Institute; American College of Cardiology Foundation; American Heart Association. Implications of recent clinical trials for the National Cholesterol Education Program Adult Treatment Panel III guidelines. *Circulation* 2004;**110**:227-39.

Yusuf S, Hawken S, Ounpuu S, Dans T, Avezum A, Lanas F, McQueen M, Budaj A, Pais P, Varigos J, Lisheng L; INTERHEART Study Investigators. Effect of potentially modifiable risk factors associated with myocardial infarction in 52 countries (the INTERHEART study): case-control study. *Lancet* 2004;**364**:937-52.

An inverse relationship between the level of HDL-C and the risk of developing premature coronary heart disease (CHD) has been consistently found in prospective population studies. In many of these studies, the level of HDL-C has been the single most powerful lipid predictor of future CHD events. Such key population studies include the Framingham Heart Study, the PROCAM Study, the Helsinki Heart Study (HHS) and the Multiple Risk Factor Intervention Trial (MRFIT).

It may be concluded from these studies that for every 1 mg/dL (0.025 mmol/L) increase in HDL-C, the risk of having a CHD event is reduced by 2-5%.

The increased CHD risk associated with a low level of HDL-C is apparent at all concentrations of LDL-C. A low level of HDL-C increases CHD risk regardless of whether the LDL-C is high, average or low, while a high level of HDL-C reduces risk even when the LDL-C is high.

The power of HDL-C as an inverse predictor of future CHD has been found in virtually every population study in which it has been investigated. Furthermore, when ranked against other known risk factors, a low level of HDL-C consistently emerges as number one, two or three.

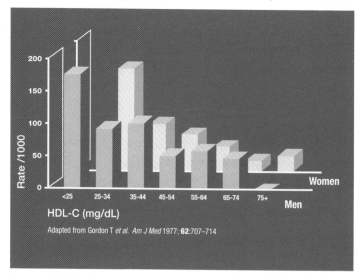

Adapted from Gordon T *et al. Am J Med* 1977; **62**:707–714

Figure II.1. HDL-C and CHD in men and women in the Framingham Heart Study

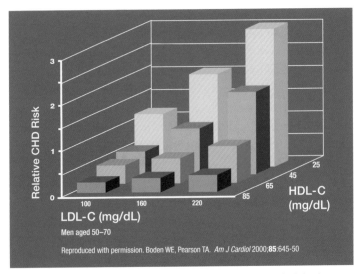

Figure II.2. HDL-C and LDL-C independent predictors of CHD in the Framingham Heart Study

HDLs and Atherosclerosis: Cause and Effect or an Epiphenomenon?

Despite the now powerful evidence that HDLs protect against atherosclerosis and that this protection is reduced in people with low HDL levels, there has been a view (now rapidly disappearing) that a low level of HDL-C is simply the reflection of some other factor or factors that are the true cause of the disease. For example, it has been argued that a low level of HDL-C is common in subjects with hypertriglyceridaemia. Since triglyceride-rich lipoproteins may be atherogenic, it has been suggested by some that the inverse relationship between the concentration of HDL-C and the development of CHD may reflect no more than the increased level of triglyceride-rich lipoproteins. Furthermore, patients with low levels of HDL-C are often obese and insulin-resistant, conditions known in their own right to be associated with an increased risk of cardiovascular disease.

However, there is also compelling evidence that a low concentration of HDL-C is a predictor of CHD, independent of LDL-C, plasma triglyceride, body weight or the presence of diabetes. Furthermore, a low level of HDL-C remains highly predictive of cardiovascular events even when the LDL-C has been reduced to very low levels by treatment with statins.

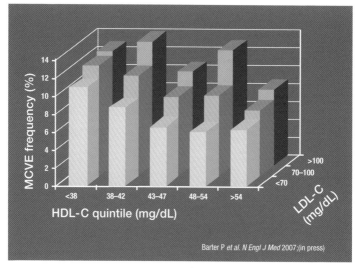

Barter P *et al. N Engl J Med* 2007;(in press)

Figure II.3. Major cardiovascular events in the TNT Trial

As described in greater detail later, there is a growing understanding of the mechanisms by which HDLs protect and evidence from basic studies in animals and intervention studies in humans that strategies to raise the concentration of HDL-C translate into a reduced risk of future cardiovascular events.

The level of HDL-C is a powerful inverse predictor of CHD.

For every 1 mg/dL (0.025 mmol/L) increase in HDL-C, the risk of having a CHD event is reduced by 2-5%.

The increased CHD risk associated with a low level of HDL-C is apparent at all concentrations of LDL-C.

Table II.1. Summary

References

Gordon T, Castelli WP, Hjortland MC, Kannel WB, Dawber TR. High density lipoprotein as a protective factor against coronary heart disease. The Framingham Study. *Am J Med* 1977;**62**:707-14.

Gordon DJ, Probstfield JL, Garrison RJ *et al*. High-density lipoprotein cholesterol and cardiovascular disease. Four prospective American studies. *Circulation* 1989;**79**:8-15.

Gordon DJ, Rifkind BM. High density lipoproteins: the clinical implications of recent studies. *N Engl J Med* 1989;**321**:1311-16.

Barter P, Kastelein J, Nunn A, Hobbs R and Future Forum Editorial Board. High density lipoproteins (HDLs) and atherosclerosis: the unanswered questions. *Atherosclerosis* 2003;**168**:195-211.

Barter P, Gotto AM, LaRosa JC *et al*., for the treating to New Targets Investigators. HDL cholesterol, very low levels of LDL cholesterol and cardiovascular events. *N Engl J Med* 2007;**357**:1301-10.

HDLs are the smallest (7.0–12 nm diameter) and densest (1.063 < d < 1.25 g/ml) of the plasma lipoproteins. They are heterogeneous, comprising several discrete subpopulations of particles that vary in shape, size, density, composition and surface charge.

Lipid-poor apoA-I   Single molecule of apoA-I   (with or without small amount of phospholipid)   *Pre-beta-migrating*
Discoidal HDL   Two or three molecules of apoA-I   (plus phospholipid with or without unesterified cholesterol)   *Pre-beta-migrating*
Spherical HDL   Two or more molecules of apoA-I   (plus phospholipid, unesterified cholesterol,   cholesteryl esters and triglyceride with or without apoA-II)   *Alpha-migrating*

Figure III.1. HDLs exist in several forms

Reproduced with permission. Rye KA, Barter PJ. *Arterioscler Thromb Vasc Biol* 2004;**24(3)**:421-8

Like the particles in other plasma lipoprotein fractions, HDLs are mostly spherical, consisting of a fatty core (in the case of HDLs this core consists mainly of cholesteryl esters with a small amount of triglyceride) surrounded by a surface layer of phospholipids, unesterified cholesterol and apolipoproteins. However, there is also a minor population of discoidal HDL particles consisting only of surface constituents arranged as a molecular bi-layer of phospholipids and unesterified cholesterol encircled by apolipoproteins.

HDL Apolipoproteins
The main apolipoproteins of HDLs are apolipoprotein (apo)A-I (about 70% of the total HDL protein) and apoA-II (about 20% of the total), although some HDL particles also contain other minor apolipoproteins such as apoA-IV, apoA-V, apoC-I, apoC-II, apoC-III, apoD, apoE, apoJ and apoL. Furthermore, HDLs transport several additional proteins, including cholesteryl ester transfer protein (CETP), lecithin:cholesterol acyltransferase (LCAT), phospholipid transfer protein (PLTP) and paraoxonase (PON).

It is interesting to note that the concentration of apoA-I in normal human subjects is more than 1.0 g/L, making it one of the most abundant proteins in human plasma.

ApoA-I	The major apolipoprotein in HDLs; accounts for about 70% of HDL protein Important function in promoting the efflux of cholesterol from cells **Activates LCAT** Has anti-oxidant and anti-inflammatory properties Most of the apoA-I in plasma exists as a component of spherical HDL particles
ApoA-II	Second most abundant protein in HDLs; accounts for about 20% of HDL protein Increases stability of the HDL particle Main function not known Most of the apoA-II in plasma exists as a component of spherical HDL particles
ApoA-IV	A minor HDL apolipoprotein Has functions very similar to apoA-I About half of the apoA-IV in plasma exists as a component of HDLs; the rest circulates in a lipid-free form
ApoA-V	A minor HDL apolipoprotein Involved more with the metabolism of triglyceride-rich lipoproteins than HDLs Most is carried in blood as a component of triglyceride-rich lipoproteins
ApoE	A minor HDL apolipoprotein Involved in cholesterol efflux from cells Plays role in recognition of HDLs (and other lipoproteins) by cell receptors Has a role in central nervous system function Most is carried in blood as a component of HDLs, with rest in triglyceride-rich lipoproteins
ApoC-I, C-II and C-III	Minor constituents of HDLs Major role in the metabolism of triglyceride-rich lipoproteins Most transported as component of triglyceride-rich lipoproteins
ApoD, apoJ, apoL & apoM	Minor components of HDLs Functions are not known

Table III.1. HDL apolipoproteins

Lecithin:cholesterol acyltransferase (LCAT)	Catalyses the esterification of cholesterol in HDL and accounts for most of the cholesteryl esters that circulate in plasma Plays major role in the metabolisms and remodelling of HDLs
Cholesteryl ester transfer protein (CETP)	Redistributes cholesteryl esters from HDLs where they are formed to other plasma lipoprotein fractions Plays major role in the metabolisms and remodelling of HDLs
Phospholipid transfer protein (PLTP)	Transfers phospholipids between HDLs and other plasma lipoprotein fractions Plays major role in the metabolisms and remodelling of HDLs
Paraoxonase (PON)	An important anti-oxidant that circulates in plasma mainly bound to HDL particles

Table III.2. Other proteins transported by HDLs

HDL Subpopulations

The HDLs circulating in human plasma comprise a number of discrete subpopulations that vary with respect to shape, size, density, apolipoprotein composition and electrophoretic mobility.

Shape

Most of the HDLs in plasma are spherical particles, although there also exists a minor subpopulation of discoidal HDLs. The discoidal particles represent a nascent form of HDLs that exist only transiently before being converted into the spherical form. The fact that the concentration of discoidal HDLs is normally very low reflects the rapidity of their conversion into spherical particles.

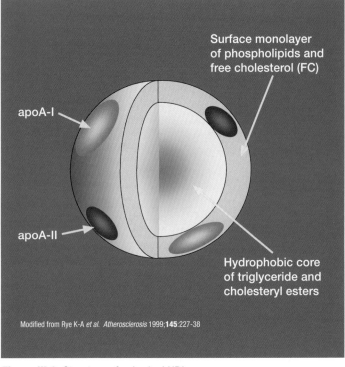

apoA-I

Surface monolayer
of phospholipids and
free cholesterol (FC)

apoA-II

Hydrophobic core
of triglyceride and
cholesteryl esters

Modified from Rye K-A *et al. Atherosclerosis* 1999;**145**:227-38

Figure III.2. Structure of spherical HDLs

Size and Density

HDLs may be separated on the basis of density into two main subfractions - HDL_2 (1.063 < d < 1.125 g/ml) and HDL_3 (1.125 < d < 1.21 g/ml) - and on the basis of particle size into five distinct subpopulations: HDL_{2b} (diameter 10.6 nm), HDL_{2a} (9.2 nm), HDL_{3a} (8.4 nm), HDL_{3b} (8.0 nm) and HDL_{3c} (7.6 nm).

Apolipoprotein Composition

HDLs may also be separated into two major subpopulations on the basis of their apolipoprotein composition. One subpopulation comprises HDLs containing apoA-I but no apoA-II (A-I HDLs), while the other comprises particles containing both apoA-I and apoA-II (A-I/A-II HDLs). ApoA-I is divided approximately equally between A-I HDLs and A-I/A-II HDLs in most subjects, while virtually all of the apoA-II resides in A-I/A-II HDLs. A small proportion of the apoA-I exists in a lipid-free or lipid-poor form.

Electrophoretic Mobility

HDLs also vary in surface charge. When separated by agarose gel electrophoresis, HDLs may have alpha, pre-beta or gamma mobility. The alpha-migrating particles tend to be spherical lipoproteins and account for the major proportion of HDLs in human plasma. Alpha-migrating HDLs include the HDL_2 and HDL_3 subfractions as well as the A-I HDL and A-I/A-II HDL subpopulations. Pre-beta HDLs are either lipid-poor (or lipid-free) apoA-I or discoidal particles consisting of one or two molecules of apoA-I complexed with phospholipids and possibly a small amount of unesterified cholesterol. Gamma-HDLs contain apoE and no apoA-I.

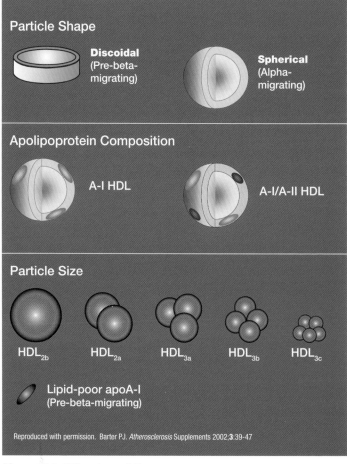

Figure III.3. HDL subpopulations

HDL Subpopulations and Atherosclerosis

It has been suggested that A-I HDLs are superior to A-I/A-II HDLs in their ability to protect against atherosclerosis, although other studies have suggested that the protection conferred by A-I HDLs and A-I/A-II HDLs is comparable. It has also been reported that larger HDLs are more protective than smaller HDLs, while others have suggested that minor subpopulations of discoidal, pre-beta-migrating HDLs are superior to spherical, alpha-migrating HDLs in their ability to inhibit atherosclerosis. Some researchers have suggested that the inverse relationship between HDL-C concentration and CHD is a function of the concentration of the HDL_2 subfraction, while others have found that the development of CHD correlates significantly and inversely with the concentrations of HDL_3 but not HDL_2.

Overall, it may be concluded that the evidence linking protection against CHD to specific HDL subpopulations in humans is conflicting and confusing. Thus, it remains unknown whether the cardioprotective effects of HDLs are influenced by their apolipoprotein composition, their size, density, electrophoretic mobility, or by a combination of all of these properties.

HDLs are the smallest and densest of the plasma lipoproteins.
The HDLs circulating in human plasma comprise a number of discrete subpopulations that vary with respect to shape, size, density, apolipoprotein composition and electrophoretic mobility.
Most HDLs in normal plasma are spherical particles.
The two main protein components of HDLs are apoA-I and apoA-II.
ApoA-I is divided approximately equally between particles that contain apoA-I without apoA-II and particles that also contain apoA-II.
ApoA-II resides only in particles that also contain apoA-I.
HDLs also transport CETP, LCAT, PLTP and paraoxonase.
It is still not known whether the cardioprotective effects of HDLs are influenced by their apolipoprotein composition, their size, density or electrophoretic mobility.

Table III.3. Summary

References

Asztalos BF, Cupples LA, Demissie S, Horvath KV, Cox CE, Batista MC, Schaefer EJ. High-density lipoprotein subpopulation profile and coronary heart disease prevalence in male participants of the Framingham Offspring Study. *Arterioscler Thromb Vasc Biol* 2004;**24**:2181-7.

Asztalos BF, Schaefer EJ. High-density lipoprotein subpopulations in pathologic conditions. *Am J Cardiol* 2003;**91**(7A):12E-17E.

Cheung MC, Albers JJ. Distribution of high density lipoprotein particles with different apoprotein composition: particles with A-I and A-II and particles with A-I but no A-II. *J Lipid Res* 1982;**23**(5):747-53.

Barter PJ, Clay MA, Rye K-A. High Density Lipoproteins: The Anti-Atherogenic Fraction. In: Plasma Lipids and their Role in Disease. Edited by Barter PJ and Rye K-A. Harwood Academic Publishers, UK, 1999;85-108.

HDLs have their origin in the liver and intestine as lipid-poor particles that acquire most of their lipid constituents after being secreted into the plasma. This is achieved in a series of reactions that culminate in the formation of mature, fully lipidated HDL particles. These reactions, and the subsequent remodelling of HDLs, are the result of activity of several factors. These include the ATP-binding cassette A1 (ABCA1), ATP-binding cassette G1 (ABCG1), scavenger receptor type B1 (SR-B1), lecithin:cholesterol acyltransferase (LCAT), cholesteryl ester transfer protein (CETP), phospholipid transfer protein (PLTP), hepatic lipase, lipoprotein lipase and endothelial lipase.

Factors Involved in the Extracellular Assembly and Remodelling of HDL

ATP-binding Cassette A1
ABCA1 is a cell membrane transporter that facilitates the delivery of cholesterol from cells to lipid-poor apoA-I in the extracellular space.

ATP-binding Cassette G1
ABCG1 is another cell membrane transporter that differs from ABCA1 in that it promotes the transfer of cholesterol from cells to large, alpha-migrating, spherical HDLs in the extracellular space.

Scavenger Receptor Type B1
SR-B1 is an HDL receptor present mainly in the liver that promotes the selective hepatic uptake of HDL cholesterol.

Lecithin:Cholesterol Acyltransferase
LCAT is a plasma protein that acts primarily on the cholesterol in HDLs. It catalyses the esterification of HDL cholesterol to form cholesteryl esters. Activity of LCAT is responsible for virtually all of the cholesteryl esters in plasma. About 80% of the cholesterol in HDLs (and 70% of that in the total plasma fraction) exists in the esterified form.

Cholesteryl Ester Transfer Protein

CETP is a plasma protein that promotes the redistribution of cholesteryl esters and triglyceride between plasma lipoproteins. The net effect of its action is a mass transfer of cholesteryl esters from HDL (where they are synthesised in the LCAT reaction) to triglyceride-rich lipoproteins in exchange for triglyceride that is transferred from triglyceride-rich lipoproteins to HDLs.

As outlined later, inhibition of CETP has been tested as a potential therapy for raising HDL levels and inhibiting atherosclerosis.

Phospholipid Transfer Protein

PLTP is plasma protein that promotes transfers of phospholipids between HDL and other plasma lipoproteins.

Hepatic Lipase

Hepatic lipase (HL) is a triglyceride lipase that resides on the surface of the endothelial cells lining hepatic sinusoids and the capillary beds of steroid hormone synthesising tissues. Its preferred substrate is HDL triglyceride.

Lipoprotein Lipase

Lipoprotein lipase (another triglyceride lipase) resides on the surface of the endothelial cells in most tissues. It hydrolyses triglyceride in chylomicrons and very low density lipoproteins (VLDLs) in a process that is accompanied by the transfer of phospholipids and apolipoproteins to HDLs.

Endothelial Lipase

Endothelial lipase (a third triglyceride lipase active in plasma) is present on the surface of all endothelial cells. Its preferred substrate is HDL phospholipid. Its precise function is still poorly understood.

These factors contribute both to the formation and the remodelling of HDLs.

Formation of A-I HDLs

ApoA-I is secreted from the liver in a lipid-free or lipid-poor form. Once in plasma it rapidly acquires phospholipids and cholesterol from cell membranes in a reaction mediated by the ABCA1 transporter that results in the formation of pre-beta-migrating, discoidal HDLs. The cholesterol in these discoidal HDLs is subsequently esterified by LCAT. The cholesteryl esters that are formed have virtually no solubility in water and cannot remain on the surface of the HDL disc where they would be in direct contact with the water plasma. Rather, they move into the inside of the particle to form a lipid core in a process that converts pre-beta-migrating HDL discs into the alpha-migrating, spherical HDL particles that predominate in plasma.

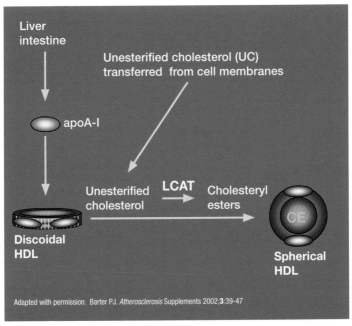

Adapted with permission. Barter PJ. *Atherosclerosis* Supplements 2002;**3**:39–47

Figure IV.1. Formation of spherical HDL

Remodelling of A-I HDLs

The spherical A-I HDLs that are formed from discoidal HDLs initially contain two molecules of apoA-I per particle. However, once formed, they are subject to extensive remodelling by plasma factors in processes that further change their composition and size. Two factors known to increase the size of spherical HDL are LCAT and PLTP. Both remodel small, alpha-migrating A-I HDL spheres into larger particles which contain three (or four) rather than two molecules of apoA-I per particle.

These larger, alpha-migrating spherical HDLs are also subject to remodelling in processes that reduce their size by depleting them of their core cholesteryl esters and triglyceride. This reduction in HDL size is accompanied by the loss of a proportion of the apoA-I from the surface of the particle.

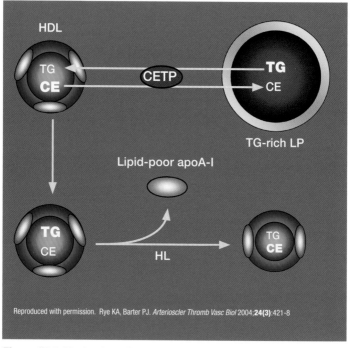

Figure IV.2. Mechanism of the remodelling of HDLs by CETP and hepatic lipase (HL)

Cycling of apoA-I Between Lipid-rich and Lipid-poor Forms

The lipid-poor apoA-I that is lost from larger HDLs during their remodelling to smaller particles may subsequently pick up new phospholipids and cholesterol from cell membranes in a process that generates new discoidal HDL particles.

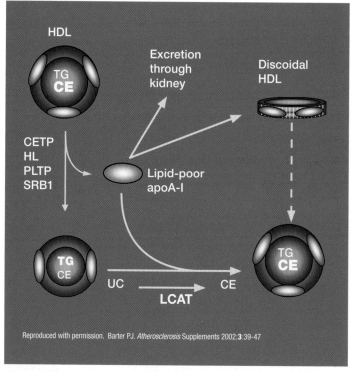

Reproduced with permission. Barter PJ. *Atherosclerosis* Supplements 2002;**3**:39-47

Figure IV.3. ApoA-I cycles between HDLs and a lipid-poor pool

Formation of A-I/A-II HDLs

Approximately half of the apoA-I in human plasma exists in spherical HDL particles that also contain apoA-II. There is compelling evidence that, like A-I HDLs, A-I/A-II HDLs are formed only after the individual components have been secreted into the plasma. ApoA-I and apoA-II enter the plasma separately and are assembled into A-I/A-II HDLs within the plasma in a fusion reaction that appears also to be dependent on LCAT.

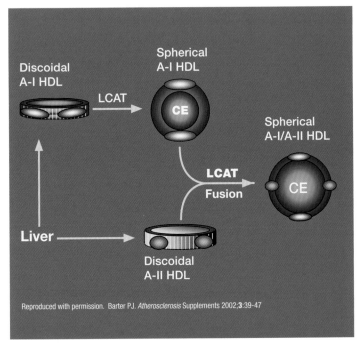

Reproduced with permission. Barter PJ. *Atherosclerosis* Supplements 2002;**3**:39-47

Figure IV.4. The role of LCAT in the formation of A-I/A-II HDLs

Plasma HDLs have their origin in the liver and intestine as lipid-poor particles that acquire most of their lipid constituents after the particle is secreted into the plasma.

After secretion into plasma, apoA-I acquires phospholipids and cholesterol from cell membranes in a process that results in the formation of discoidal A-I HDLs.

The cholesterol in discoidal HDLs is subsequently esterified in a process that converts the HDL discs into the spherical HDL particles that predominate in plasma.

Spherical A-I HDLs are subject to extensive remodelling by plasma factors in processes that further change their composition and size.

Spherical A-I/A-II HDLs (the other main HDL subpopulation) are formed within the plasma by the fusion of A-I HDLs and A-II HDLs.

Table IV.1. Summary

References

Barter PJ. The regulation and remodelling of HDL by plasma factors. *Atherosclerosis* Supplements 2002;**3**:39-47.

Rye K-A, Clay MA, Barter PJ. Remodelling of high density lipoproteins by plasma factors. *Atherosclerosis* 1999;**145**:227-38.

Rye K-A, Barter PJ. Formation and metabolism of prebeta-migrating, lipid-poor apolipoprotein A-I. *Arterioscler Thromb Vasc Biol* 2004;**24**:421-8.

Wang N, Lan D, Chen W *et al*. ATP-binding cassette transporters G1 and G4 mediate cellular cholesterol efflux to high-density lipoproteins. *Proc Natl Acad Sci USA* 2004;**101**:9774-9.

Lee JY, Parks JS. ATP-binding cassette transporter AI and its role in HDL formation. *Curr Opin Lipidol* 2005;**16**:19-25.

HDLs may be regulated both at the level of their synthesis and their catabolism.

Synthesis

An increase in synthesis of apoA-I results in an increased concentration of A-I HDLs in plasma, while an increase in apoA-II synthesis increases the plasma concentration of A-I/A-II HDLs. However, the precise regulation of the synthesis of these apolipoproteins is still poorly understood. As outlined later, drugs such as fibrates, statins and niacin all increase the synthesis of these apolipoproteins, although probably by different (and still poorly defined) mechanisms.

Catabolism

Removal of HDLs from plasma is complex, with most constituents being removed separately rather than as a part of the intact particle. For example, HDL cholesteryl esters may be transferred to VLDLs and LDLs by CETP and removed from plasma as a component of these lipoproteins. Alternatively, HDL cholesteryl esters may be selectively taken up by the liver or steroidogenic tissues in a process dependent on the binding of HDLs to SR-B1. HDL, triglyceride and phospholipids are removed by a process of hydrolysis catalysed by hepatic lipase, lipoprotein lipase, endothelial lipase and, possibly, also by secretory phospholipase A2 (sPLA2). The apoA-I in HDL is also independently metabolised following its dissociation from the particle during HDL remodelling. Regulation of the catabolism of HDLs is therefore secondary to the regulation of the complex series of reactions involved in HDL remodelling in plasma.

HDL levels are regulated by factors that regulate both synthesis and catabolism
Synthesis
• Synthesis of apoA-I is the main determinant of the concentration of A-I HDLs. • Synthesis of apoA-II is the main determinant of the concentration of A-I/A-II HDLs.
Catabolism
• Individual constituents of HDLs are removed from plasma separately rather than as a part of an uptake of the intact particle. • Regulation of the catabolism of HDLs is secondary to the regulation of reactions involved in HDL remodelling in plasma.

Table V.1. Summary

References

Rader DJ, Castro G, Zech LA, Fruchart JC, Brewer HB Jr. In vivo metabolism of apolipoprotein A-I on high density lipoprotein particles LpA-I and LpA-I, A-II. *J Lipid Res* 1991;**32**:1849-59.

Ikewaki K, Zech LA, Kindt M, Brewer HB Jr, Rader DJ. Apolipoprotein A-II production rate is a major factor regulating the distribution of apolipoprotein A-I among HDL subclasses LpA-I and LpA-I:A-II in normolipidemic humans. *Arterioscler Thromb Vasc Biol* 1995;**15**:306-31.

The functions of HDLs may be divided into two categories: those involved in plasma cholesterol transport and those that may be unrelated to cholesterol transport. Each of these categories will be described separately.

Role of HDLs in Plasma Cholesterol Transport

In order to understand the cholesterol transport functions of HDLs, it is necessary to see where they fit in to the overall scheme of cholesterol transport in plasma.

Transport of Dietary Cholesterol from Intestine to Liver

Dietary cholesterol is absorbed by intestinal cells where it becomes esterified (by an enzyme known as acyl-coenzyme A:cholesterol acyltransferase or ACAT) before being incorporated (with triglyceride) into chylomicrons. Chylomicrons are then secreted into intestinal lymph ducts and eventually transported to the blood plasma via the thoracic duct in a process that may take as long as 10 hours after completing the meal.

Once in plasma, chylomicrons are rapidly metabolised by lipoprotein lipase (LPL) that breaks down their triglyceride, releasing free fatty acids (FFA) as a source of energy or stored fat. The loss of triglyceride results in the conversion of the chylomicron into a smaller chylomicron remnant particle that then delivers dietary cholesterol to the liver.

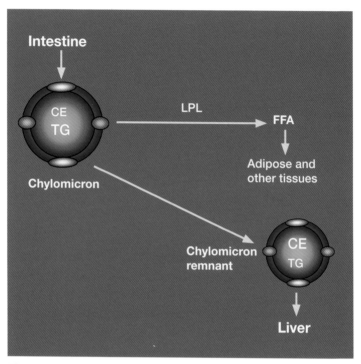

Figure VI.1. Transport of cholesterol from diet to liver

Transport of Cholesterol from Liver to Extrahepatic Tissues

In addition to receiving dietary cholesterol (as delivered by chylomicron remnants) the liver also synthesises its own cholesterol. Hepatic cholesterol, whether from the diet or newly synthesised, may be used for several purposes, including membrane synthesis, conversion into bile acids or incorporation (with triglyceride) into VLDLs. The VLDLs (and the cholesterol they contain) are subsequently secreted into plasma where their triglyceride is broken down by lipoprotein lipase, releasing free fatty acids for uptake by tissues. As it loses its triglyceride, the VLDL particle becomes progressively smaller and, in a complex series of reactions, is ultimately converted into a triglyceride-poor, cholesterol-rich LDL particle.

The cholesterol in LDLs is subsequently delivered to tissues following binding of the particles to LDL receptors. Since the level of expression of the LDL receptor is increased in cells that are depleted of cholesterol and decreased in cells that are overloaded with cholesterol, this process ensures that the cholesterol in LDLs is delivered precisely where it is needed, whether this is a return of the cholesterol to the liver or an uptake of cholesterol by cells in extrahepatic tissues.

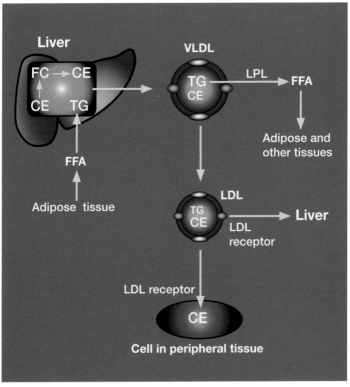

Figure VI.2. Transport of cholesterol from liver to cells

Transport of Cholesterol from Extrahepatic Tissues to the Liver: Reverse Cholesterol Transport

Only the liver and endocrine tissues that synthesise steroid hormones have the ability to metabolise the cholesterol molecule. Other tissues are totally dependent on an efflux to acceptors in the extracellular space to remove their surplus cholesterol. The predominant extracellular acceptors are HDLs.

There are at least four distinct processes that promote the efflux of cholesterol from cells. One involves activity of ABCA1, with lipid-free apoA-I acting as the main acceptor. A second involves ABCG1, with large spherical HDL acting as the main acceptor. A third involves SR-B1 (again with large spherical HDL as the main acceptor). There is also a fourth process that involves passive diffusion of cholesterol from cell membranes to HDL particles in the extracellular space. The relative importance of these four processes is uncertain and may vary between different cell types and under different physiological circumstances.

ABCA1 promotes a net efflux of cholesterol from cells to lipid-free apoA-I in the extracellular space.
ABCG1 promotes a net efflux of cholesterol from cells (including macrophages) to large, spherical HDL particles in the extracellular space.
SR-B1 mediates a bidirectional transfer of cholesterol between cells and spherical HDLs. It promotes a net efflux of cholesterol only if there is a concentration gradient of cholesterol from the donor cell to the acceptor HDL. Such a concentration gradient is generated by the LCAT-mediated esterification of cholesterol on the surface of HDL particles.
Passive Diffusion of cholesterol to spherical HDLs also occurs. This results in an exchange of cholesterol between HDLs and cell membranes. A net efflux of cholesterol into HDLs depends on the presence of an LCAT-mediated concentration gradient from the cell to the HDL particle.

Table VI.1. Summary of the main efflux processes

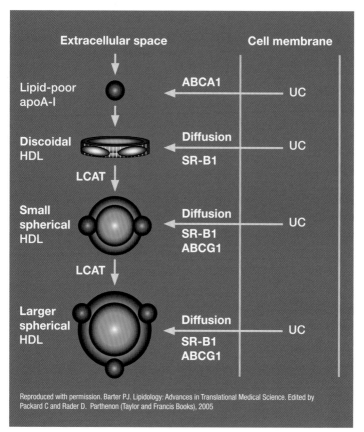

Figure VI.3. Four processes that promote efflux of cholesterol from cells to HDLs

Once the cholesterol has been transferred from cells to HDLs in the extracellular space, it may be delivered to the liver for elimination from the body by either direct or indirect pathways.

It may be delivered directly to the liver in a process involving binding of HDLs to SR-B1. Alternatively, it may be delivered to the liver by an indirect pathway involving the CETP-mediated transfer of HDL cholesteryl esters to the VLDL/LDL fraction, with delivery to the liver then being achieved by the receptor-mediated uptake of LDLs.

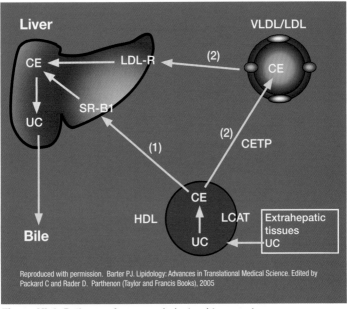

Reproduced with permission. Barter PJ. Lipidology: Advances in Translational Medical Science. Edited by Packard C and Rader D. Parthenon (Taylor and Francis Books), 2005

Figure VI.4. Pathway of reverse cholesterol transport

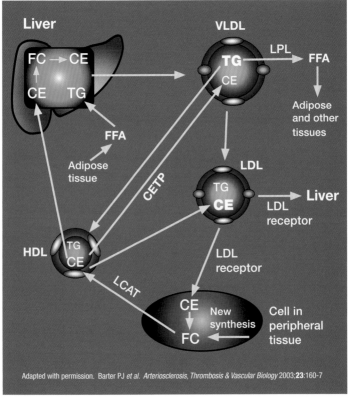

Adapted with permission. Barter PJ *et al. Arteriosclerosis, Thrombosis & Vascular Biology* 2003;**23**:160-7

Figure VI.5. Overview of plasma cholesterol transport

Non-lipid Functions of HDLs
In addition to their well-known role in plasma cholesterol transport, HDLs also have a number of other functions, some of which may contribute substantially to their anti-atherogenic properties.

Anti-oxidant Properties of HDLs
HDLs inhibit the formation of potentially atherogenic oxidised LDLs. This may be achieved either by the paraoxonase that is transported by HDLs or by apolipoproteins such as apoA-I, apoA-II, apoA-IV and apoE, all of which have anti-oxidant properties.

Anti-inflammatory Properties of HDLs
HDLs inhibit the expression of the adhesion proteins, VCAM-1, ICAM-1 and E-selectin, in endothelial cells. These adhesion proteins are fundamental to the recruitment of monocytes into the artery wall in the early stages of atherosclerosis.

Anti-thrombotic Properties of HDLs
HDLs inhibit the expression of pro-thrombotic tissue factor by endothelial cells.

Endothelial Stabilising Properties of HDLs
HDLs have been shown to normalise endothelial function in patients with either low HDL levels or high LDL levels.

Endothelial Repair Properties of HDLs
HDLs promote the repair of damaged endothelium.

Anti-oxidant
Anti-inflammatory
Anti-thrombotic
Endothelial stabilisation
Endothelial repair

Table VI.2. Non-lipid functions of HDLs

Cholesterol transport functions

A major role of HDLs in plasma cholesterol transport is to deliver cholesterol from extrahepatic tissues to the liver for recycling or for elimination from the body in bile.

Non-lipid functions of HDLs

In addition to their role in plasma cholesterol transport, HDLs also have other potentially anti-atherogenic properties:

- Anti-oxidant
- Anti-inflammatory
- Anti-thrombotic
- Endothelial stabilising

Table VI.3. Summary

References

Fielding CJ, Fielding PE. Molecular physiology of reverse cholesterol transport. *J Lipid Res* 1995;**36**:211-28.

Barter PJ, Nicholls SJ, Rye K-A, Anantharamaiah GM, Navab M, Fogelman AM. Anti-inflammatory properties of HDL. *Circ Res* 2004;**95**:764-72.

O'Connell BJ, Genest J Jr. High-density lipoproteins and endothelial function. *Circulation* 2001;**104**:1978-83.

In order to understand how HDLs protect against atherosclerosis, it is first necessary to understand what causes the atherosclerosis in the first place.

Role of Atherogenic Lipoproteins in Causing Atherosclerosis

Atherosclerosis is an inflammatory disorder caused by the accumulation of atherogenic lipoproteins in the artery wall. LDLs are the main atherogenic lipoproteins in plasma, although the catabolic remnants of chylomicrons and VLDLs have also been implicated in the development of atherosclerosis.

The initiating event is the incorporation of an atherogenic lipoprotein into the artery wall. LDLs, chylomicron remnants and VLDL remnants all cross the endothelial lining and enter the subendothelial space. They may also return from the artery wall to the plasma. However, if the plasma concentration is above a threshold level (the precise threshold is not known), the rate of entry exceeds removal and the particles accumulate in the artery wall. As they accumulate, they become modified in various ways. The best-known modification is oxidation. Oxidised LDLs or remnants then initiate a series of events that culminate in the development of atherosclerosis.

The subsequent discussion will refer to LDLs but also applies to the remnants of triglyceride-rich lipoproteins.

Oxidised LDLs stimulate endothelial cells to express monocyte chemotactic protein-1 (MCP-1), a chemokine that attracts monocytes from blood into the artery wall. The oxidised LDLs then promote differentiation of these monocytes into macrophages within the artery wall. The macrophages express scavenger receptors capable of binding and taking up the oxidised LDLs. The resulting cellular accumulation of cholesterol leads to the formation of foam cells, the hallmark cell of developing atherosclerosis.

Macrophages and foam cells secrete growth factors that lead to cell proliferation and proteinases that break down the matrix of the vessel wall. These processes lead ultimately to the development of advanced, complicated, rupture-prone atherosclerotic plaques.

Macrophages in the artery wall also secrete cytokines, including tumour necrosis factor (TNF)-α and interleukin-1, that stimulate endothelial cells to express the adhesion proteins, vascular cell adhesion molecule-1 (VCAM-1), intercellular adhesion molecule-1 (ICAM-1) and E-selectin. These adhesion proteins bind blood monocytes, making them accessible for recruitment into the artery wall by MCP-1, thus creating a vicious cycle that greatly amplifies the effects of the modified LDLs.

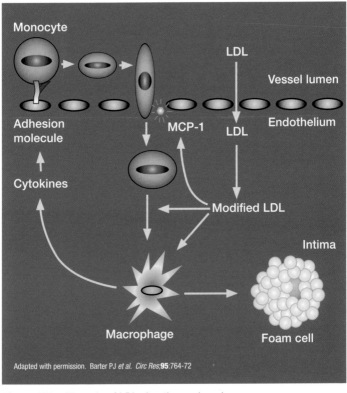

Adapted with permission. Barter PJ *et al. Circ Res*;**95**:764-72

Figure VII.1. The role of LDLs in atherosclerosis

Role of HDLs in Protecting against Atherosclerosis

HDLs have the ability to protect against atherosclerosis by several mechanisms.

The best known mechanism relates to their ability to promote the efflux of cholesterol from foam cells, thus inhibiting the progression (and even promoting the regression) of atherosclerosis.

HDLs also inhibit the oxidative modification of the LDLs and thus reduce their atherogenicity.

HDLs inhibit the expression of endothelial cell adhesion molecules and MCP-1.

In addition, HDLs are anti-thrombotic. They also stimulate the generation of nitric oxide, thus reducing the endothelial dysfunction that may precede the development of atherosclerosis.

And recently, HDLs have been shown to promote the repair of damaged endothelium.

HDLs, therefore, have several properties that contribute to their ability to protect against the development of atherosclerosis.

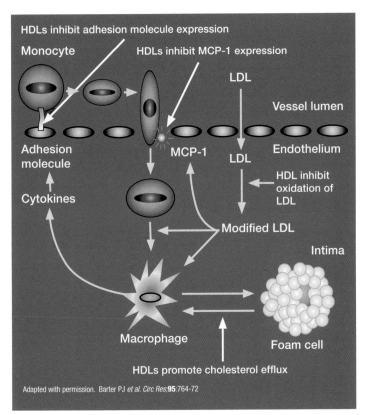

Figure VII.2. Inhibition of atherosclerosis by HDLs

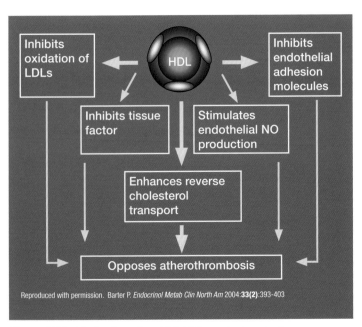

Figure VII.3. Mechanisms by which HDLs protect against atherosclerosis

Atherosclerosis is an inflammatory disorder caused by the accumulation of atherogenic lipoproteins in the artery wall.
LDLs and the catabolic remnants of chylomicrons and VLDLs are the main atherogenic lipoproteins in plasma.
The initiating event is the incorporation of an atherogenic lipoprotein into the artery wall followed by a cascade of events that culminates in the development of an atherosclerotic plaque.
HDLs protect against atherosclerosis by several mechanisms, including promotion of the efflux of cholesterol from foam cells, inhibition of the oxidative modification of atherogenic lipoproteins, inhibition of vascular inflammation and inhibition of thrombosis.

Table VII.1. Summary

References

Ross R. The pathogenesis of atherosclerosis: a perspective for the 1990s. *Nature* 1993;**362**:801-09.

Barter PJ, Rye K-A. High density lipoproteins and coronary heart disease. *Atherosclerosis* 1996;**121**:1-12.

Assman G, Nofer J-R. Atheroprotective effects of high density lipoproteins. *Ann Rev Med* 2003;**54**:321-41.

Calebresi L *et al*. Endotheleial protection by high density lipoproteins. *Arterioscler Thromb Vasc Biol* 2003;**23**:1724-31.

Protection against Atherosclerosis

Studies in Animals

HDLs have been shown to have direct anti-atherogenic properties in a range of studies in animals. These include the infusion of HDL into cholesterol-fed rabbits and the over-expression of apoA-I in transgenic rabbits and mice.

What about Humans?

Despite the very large body of epidemiological evidence identifying HDL-C as a powerful negative risk factor in humans, there are very few intervention studies that have put this proposition directly to the test. While there are several human intervention studies in which drug-induced elevations of HDL-C are associated with a reduction in atherosclerosis (see chapters XI, XII and XIII), most of these trials were not designed specifically to test the benefits of raising the level of HDL-C.

There are, however, two direct studies in humans that provide strong support for the proposition that raising the level of HDLs is of substantial therapeutic advantage.

One was a small study in which a preparation of reconstituted HDLs was infused into human subjects with coronary artery disease. The HDL contained a variant of apoA-I (known as apoA-I$_{Milano}$) complexed with a phospholipid. Subjects received intravenous injections of the HDL preparation at weekly intervals for just five weeks. This resulted in a significant reduction in the atheroma burden in the coronary arteries as assessed by intravascular ultrasound. While the study included only a small number of subjects, the result was consistent with a profound protective action of HDL and provided a powerful incentive to conduct further research.

A second larger study also used reconstituted HDLs but in this case the HDLs were prepared from normal apoA-I. Patients were randomly assigned to receive four weekly infusions of either saline or the reconstituted HDLs. In this study, infusion of reconstituted HDLs had no significant effect on percentage change in coronary atheroma volume (as assessed by intravascular ultrasound) compared with placebo but did result in statistically significant improvement in the plaque characterisation index and coronary score as assessed by quantitative coronary angiography.

Patients received five weekly infusions of placebo or a complex containing apoA-I$_{Milano}$ and phospholipids.
Intravascular ultrasound was performed within two weeks following ACS and repeated after five weekly treatments.
The primary efficacy parameter was the change in percent atheroma volume.
Mean atheroma volume decreased significantly by -1.06% (p =.02) in the treated group compared with a 0.14% increase in atheroma volume in the placebo group.

Table VIII.1. Effect of recombinant apoA-I$_{Milano}$ on coronary atherosclerosis

Protection by HDLs against Acute Inflammation in Stroke, Acute Coronary Syndromes and Endotoxic Shock

There is mounting evidence that anti-inflammatory properties of HDLs may offer therapeutic benefits beyond their ability to protect against atherosclerosis. For example, it has been shown in studies of experimental stroke in rats that pre-treatment with HDLs significantly and substantially reduces the brain necrotic area. Furthermore, in a study of haemorrhagic shock in rats, the resulting multiple organ dysfunction syndrome was largely abolished by a single injection of human HDLs given 90 minutes after the haemorrhage. In that model, injection of HDLs prevented both the severe disruption of tissue architecture and the extensive cellular infiltration into the affected tissues. Intravenous infusions of relatively small amounts of reconstituted HDLs have also been shown to markedly reduce the acute vascular inflammation induced by the application of a non-occlusive collar to carotid arteries of rabbits.

Thus, it is apparent that HDLs have acute anti-inflammatory effects that are extremely rapid and possibly unrelated to the cholesterol transport function

of these lipoproteins. Such properties of HDLs have
implications beyond their documented ability to protect
against atherosclerosis and suggest a potential role
of HDLs in the management of acute inflammatory
states such as acute coronary syndromes, stroke and
ischaemia-reperfusion injury.

HDLs promote regression of atherosclerosis in animals.
While human intervention studies are consistent with the protective role of HDLs, most trials have not been designed to test the benefits of HDL raising.
In one small study in humans, intravenous infusion of a preparation of reconstituted HDLs over a period of five weeks promoted a significant reduction in coronary atheroma burden.
Infusion of HDLs reduces the tissue damage in brain in experimental stroke in rats.

Table VIII.2. Summary

References

Badimon JJ, Badimon L, Fuster V. Regression of atherosclerotic lesions
by high density lipoprotein plasma traction in the cholesterol-fed rabbit.
J Clin Invest 1990;**85**:1234-41.

Rubin EM, Krauss RM, Spangler EA *et al*. Inhibition of early
atherogenesis in transgenic mice by human apolipoprotein AI. *Nature*
1991;**53**:265-7.

Plump AS, Scott CJ, Breslow J. Human apolipoprotein A-I gene
expression increases high density lipoprotein and suppresses
atherosclerosis in the apolipoprotein E-deficient mouse. *Proc Natl Acad
Sci USA* 1994;**91**:9607-11.

Duverger N, Kruth H, Emmanuel F *et al*. Inhibition of atherosclerosis
development in cholesterol-fed human apolipoprotein A-I-transgenic
rabbits. *Circulation* 1996;**94**:713-17.

Nissen SE, Tsunoda T, Tuzcu EM, Schoenhagen P, Cooper CJ,
Yasin M, Eaton GM, Lauer MA, Sheldon WS, Grines CL, Halpern S,
Crowe T, Blankenship JC, Kerensky R. Effect of recombinant ApoA-I
Milano on coronary atherosclerosis in patients with acute coronary
syndromes: a randomised controlled trial. *JAMA* 2003;**290**:2292-300.

Paterno R, Ruocco A, Postiglione A, Hubsch A, Andresen I, Lang MG.
Reconstituted high-density lipoprotein exhibits neuroprotection in two
rat models of stroke. *Cerebrovasc Dis* 2004;**17**:204-11.

Nicholls SJ, Drummond GR, Rye K-A, Dusting GJ, Barter PJ.
Reconstituted high density lipoproteins inhibit the pro-oxidant and
proinflammatory vascular changes induced by a periarterial collar in
normocholesterolemic rabbits. *Circulation* 2005;**111**:1543-50.

9 What are the Causes of Low HDL-C in Humans?

Two disorders account for the majority of cases of low HDL-C in humans: type 2 diabetes and the metabolic syndrome. Both of these conditions are approaching epidemic proportions worldwide. Less common causes include genetic conditions such as ABCA1 deficiency, deficiencies of HDL apolipoproteins, lipoprotein lipase deficiency and LCAT deficiency. Low levels of HDL-C may also accompany other dyslipidaemic states such as familial combined hyperlipidaemia and familial hypertriglyceridaemia. However, it is the low HDL associated with diabetes and the metabolic syndrome that accounts for the overwhelming majority of people with low levels of HDL-C and which provides the major stimulus for regarding HDLs as a major therapeutic target for the prevention and treatment of atherosclerosis.

| Isolated low HDL: Genetic |
| Familial combined hyperlipidaemia |
| Elevated plasma triglyceride |
| Type 2 diabetes mellitus |
| Metabolic syndrome |

Table IX.1. Causes of low HDL-C in humans

The metabolic syndrome is a cluster of abnormalities that define a condition with high cardiovascular risk. The components of the syndrome include central obesity, insulin resistance, dyslipidaemia, mild hypertension and a pro-inflammatory state. The relationship of the metabolic syndrome to type 2 diabetes is not known, although the co-existence of the two conditions in some families suggests that there is a link. Some consider the metabolic syndrome to be a pre-diabetic state.

Abdominal obesity
Insulin resistance
Elevated plasma triglyceride
Low HDL-C
Small, dense LDL
Pro-inflammatory state
Elevated free fatty acids
Mild hypertension

Table IX.2. Features of the metabolic syndrome

Dyslipidaemia in Type 2 Diabetes and the Metabolic Syndrome

The lipid abnormalities in type 2 diabetes and the metabolic syndrome are remarkably similar. They include an increased level of plasma triglyceride, an LDL fraction characterised by small, dense particles, a decreased level of HDL-C and an HDL fraction characterised by small, dense particles.

Increased plasma and VLDL triglyceride
LDL fraction characterised by small, dense particles
Increased plasma free fatty acids
Decreased HDL cholesterol
HDL fraction characterised by small, dense particles

Table IX.3. Typical dyslipidaemia in type 2 diabetes and metabolic syndrome

Mechanism of the Low HDL-C level in Type 2 Diabetes and the Metabolic Syndrome

The low level of HDL-C in people with type 2 diabetes or the metabolic syndrome is caused mainly by an increased rate of HDL catabolism, possibly secondary to triglyceride enrichment of the particles.

The most likely sequence of events is as follows:
(i) there is an increase in concentration of triglyceride-rich lipoproteins (TGR-LP); (ii) in the presence of CETP, the increased pool of triglyceride-rich lipoproteins leads to an increase in the transfer of cholesteryl esters from HDLs to the triglyceride-rich lipoproteins in exchange for triglyceride; (iii) this generates HDLs that are depleted of cholesteryl esters and enriched in triglyceride; (iv) the triglyceride enrichment provides HDLs with the preferred substrate for hepatic lipase. Subsequent hydrolysis of the newly acquired HDL triglyceride by hepatic lipase leads to a reduction in volume of the particle core, a consequent decrease in particle size and a dissociation of lipid-free/lipid-poor apoA-I from the HDL particle surface.

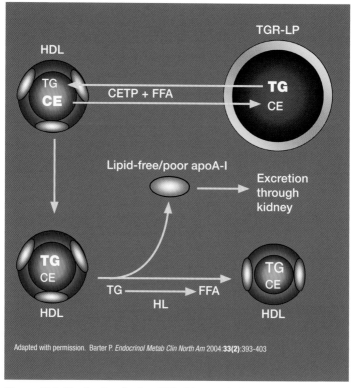

Adapted with permission. Barter P. *Endocrinol Metab Clin North Am* 2004:**33(2)**:393-403

Figure IX.1. Mechanism for low HDL-C in type 2 diabetes and the metabolic syndrome

Type 2 diabetes and the metabolic syndrome account for the majority of cases of low HDL-C in humans.

The metabolic syndrome is a cluster of abnormalities that includes central obesity, insulin resistance, dyslipidaemia, mild hypertension and a pro-inflammatory state.

The lipid abnormalities in type 2 diabetes and the metabolic syndrome are similar and characterised by an increased level of plasma triglyceride, an LDL fraction containing small, dense particles, a decreased level of HDL-C and an HDL fraction characterised by small, dense particles.

The low level of HDL-C in people with type 2 diabetes or the metabolic syndrome is caused mainly by an increased rate of HDL catabolism.

Table IX.4. Summary

References

Ginsberg HN. Insulin resistance and cardiovascular disease. *J Clin Invest* 2000;**287**:356-9.

Barter P. Metabolic abnormalities: high-density lipoproteins. *Endocrinol Metab Clin North Am* 2004;**33**:393-403.

Krauss RM. Lipids and lipoproteins in patients with type 2 diabetes. *Diabetes Care* 2004;**27**:1496-504.

Composition of the Diet

When compared with carbohydrate, dietary fats increase the concentration of HDL-C, with the effect of dietary saturated fat being greater than that of unsaturated fat. The HDL-C response to diets rich in monounsaturated and polyunsaturated (both omega-3 and omega-6) fats is comparable. Dietary cholesterol also increases the level of HDL-C. The precise mechanism by which dietary fat and cholesterol increase HDL levels is largely unknown. Nor is it known whether the increase in concentration of HDL-C induced by fat or cholesterol is beneficial. In the case of saturated fat and cholesterol in the diet, any benefits arising from an increase in HDL-C may be more than outweighed by the known detrimental effects of an accompanying increase in cholesterol in the VLDL-LDL fractions.

Weight Reduction

Many (although not all) overweight people have a low level of HDL-C. Weight reduction is usually accompanied by an increase in the HDL-C level, although to be effective, the weight loss needs to be substantial and sustained. The mechanism underlying a relationship between body weight and HDL-C concentration is uncertain, although in most cases the low HDL is present as a component of the metabolic syndrome.

Physical Activity

High levels of aerobic activity are associated with high levels of HDL-C, especially of the HDL_2 subfraction. Furthermore, increasing the level of physical activity in people with low levels of HDL-C, especially in those who are overweight, usually increases the HDL-C concentration. There is evidence that exercise increases HDL-C in part by stimulating lipoprotein lipase activity.

It has been argued that the single most important preventable cause of low HDL-C in the 21st century is a low level of physical activity.

A recent meta-analysis has confirmed the benefit of regular aerobic exercise on raising HDL-C levels and provided some insights into how much exercise is required. The analysis included 25 randomised controlled studies that were designed to evaluate the effect of exercise training on HDL-C levels. Overall, the mean exercise-induced increase in HDL-C was 2.53 mg/dL (p<0.001). Importantly, an increase in HDL-C concentration was apparent only in people who expended at least 900 kcal or exercised for at least 120 minutes each week. In these people, every 10 minutes prolongation of exercise per session was associated with a 1.4 mg/dL increase in HDL-C. In further analyses it was found that the increase in HDL-C was greatest in people whose body mass index was < 28 kg/m^2 and whose total plasma cholesterol concentration was at least 220 mg/dL (5.7 mmol/L).

These findings re-enforce recommendations for increasing levels of activity as a cardioprotective strategy but suggest that there may be substantial additional benefits of exercising for more than the currently recommended 30 minutes per day of moderate-intensity exercise.

Alcohol
Alcohol consumption increases the level of HDL-C, with most evidence favouring a selective increase in the HDL$_3$ subfraction. Alcohol has been reported to inhibit CETP, although this has not been a consistent finding and the precise mechanism by which alcohol influences HDL-C levels is not known. Nor is it known whether the HDL-C elevation associated with alcohol consumption contributes to a possible cardioprotective effect of alcohol.

Smoking Cessation
Smoking reduces the concentration of HDL-C and smoking cessation is associated with an up to 10% increase in HDL-C level. The mechanism and impact on CHD of smoking-mediated effects on HDLs are not known.

Composition of the diet
Weight reduction
Increased physical activity
Alcohol consumption
Smoking cessation

Table X.1. Lifestyle modifications that raise the level of HDL-C

Pharmacological Management

Levels of HDL-C are increased by treatment with several classes of currently available lipid-modifying agents. These include fibrates, statins and (especially) niacin, with evidence accumulating that such increases do translate into a reduced risk of cardiovascular disease. LDL-C lowering agents, such as bile acid sequestering resins (cholestyramine and colestipol) and cholesterol absorption inhibitors (ezetimibe), may also increase the level of HDL-C but the magnitude of the effect is very small and probably of little clinical importance. The effects of fibrates, statins and niacin are described in detail in the next three chapters.

Fibrates increase HDL-C by 20%
Statins increase HDL-C by 5-10%
Niacin increases HDL-C by up to 30%

Table X.2. HDL raising drugs

References
Kodama S, Tanaka S, Saito K *et al*. Effect of aerobic exercise training on serum levels of high-density lipoprotein cholesterol: a meta-analysis. *Arch Intern Med* 2007;**167**:999-1008.

Fibrates increase HDL-C by 20%. They also lower plasma triglyceride by up to 50%. The magnitude of the HDL-C increase is greatest in those individuals with lower baseline levels. Fibrates increase the concentration of both the main HDL apolipoproteins, apoA-I and apoA-II, although the effect on apoA-II often exceeds that on apoA-I.

Mode of Action of Fibrates

Fibrates work by activating the nuclear transcription factor, peroxisome proliferator-activated receptor α (PPARα). PPARs belong to the family of hormone-activated nuclear receptors. PPARα activators impact on the concentration of HDL-C by several mechanisms. They increase the synthesis of apoA-I, apoA-II, lipoprotein lipase and ABCA1. These effects all contribute to the elevation of HDL levels. Fibrate-induced activation of PPARα also increases the synthesis of SR-B1. This increases the selective hepatic uptake of HDL cholesteryl esters and thus tends to reduce the level of HDL-C. The influence of fibrates on HDL-C concentration is therefore the net effect of several factors.

Because of their opposing effects, the fibrate-induced increases in SR-B1 and ABCA1 may neutralise each other and have no net effect on HDL-C concentration. Despite this, increases in ABCA1 and SR-B1 both have the capacity to increase reverse cholesterol transport. Thus, fibrates may enhance the anti-atherogenic function of HDLs to a greater extent than would be suggested by the magnitude of the increase in HDL-C concentration.

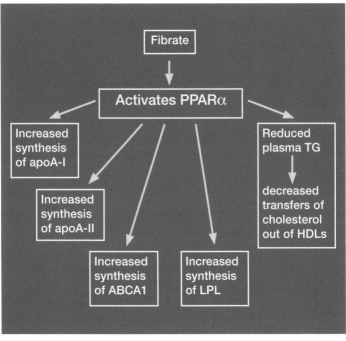

Figure XI.1. HDL raising effects of fibrates

Adverse Effects of Fibrates

Fibrates are generally very well tolerated. Reported adverse effects are mainly gastrointestinal in nature and are mostly mild and transient. Other reported effects include headache, anxiety, vertigo, dizziness, sleep disorders, arthralgia, rash, pruritus, urticaria and blurred vision. A small increase in risk of developing gallstones has also been reported, as has an increase in plasma transaminase levels. A small increase in risk of pancreatitis has also been described. Fibrates are contraindicated in people with severe hepatic dysfunction or with diseases of the gallbladder. Fibrates are well tolerated in people with diabetes, renal failure and renal transplants. Myositis is a rare adverse effect, although this tends to occur more with gemfibrozil than with other fibrates and even then only when it is co-administered with a statin.

Fenofibrate results in an increase in the concentration of plasma homocysteine, although the clinical significance is not known. A small increase in serum creatinine may also occur in people taking fenofibrate, although this does not appear to reflect renal damage. The increase is not progressive and is generally reversed if the drug is stopped.

Mild and transient gastrointestinal disturbances
Slight increase in risk of gallstones
Small increase in risk of pancreatitis
Small increase in the concentration of plasma homocysteine
Myositis (rare); tends to occur more with gemfibrozil than with other fibrates, especially if co-administered with a statin

Table XI.1. Adverse effects of fibrates

Clinical Relevance of HDL-C Raising by Fibrates

Clinical Trials with Fibrates

There have been several clinical trials investigating the effects of fibrates on cardiovascular events.

The WHO clofibrate study was an early, double-blind, placebo-controlled trial in which clofibrate was used as the active agent in individuals who were predominantly hypercholesterolaemic. CHD events were reduced from 7.4% in the placebo group to 5.9% in the clofibrate group (p<0.05). There was also a small (but significant) excess of non-coronary deaths in the group receiving clofibrate, an observation that led many to be cautious about the continued use of this drug class. It should be emphasised, however, that subsequent re-analysis of the data on the more appropriate "intention-to-treat basis" showed that the increase in non-CHD deaths was not significant. It is relevant that subsequent trials with other fibrates (with gemfibrozil in the HHS and VA-HIT study and with bezafibrate in the BIP study) have not observed a significant excess of non-coronary deaths.

The Helsinki Heart Study (HHS) was a five-year, double-blind, placebo-controlled trial in 4081 men aged 40-55 years who were free of clinically manifest CHD at entry to the study. The active treatment was gemfibrozil

1200 mg per day. The mean baseline lipid levels were: serum total cholesterol 270 mg/dL (7.0 mmol/L), LDL-C 190 mg/dL (4.9 mmol/L), HDL-C 47 mg/dL (1.22 mmol/L) and serum triglyceride 177 mg/dL (2.0 mmol/L).

Gemfibrozil increased the concentration of HDL-C by 11% and decreased the levels of serum total cholesterol, LDL-C and serum triglyceride by 10%, 11% and 35%, respectively. These lipid changes were associated with a statistically significant 34.0% reduction in the incidence of total coronary events (non-fatal myocardial infarction, fatal myocardial infarction, sudden cardiac death or unwitnessed death) from 41.4 per 1000 in the placebo group to 27.3 per 1000 in the gemfibrozil group.

The Veterans Affairs High-Density Lipoprotein Intervention Trial (VA-HIT) was designed to test the hypothesis that raising the concentration of HDL-C by treatment with gemfibrozil protects against CHD events. This study was a five-year, double-blind, placebo-controlled trial that included 2531 men aged < 74 years with known clinical CHD. It was conducted in people with low levels of both HDL-C and LDL-C. The active treatment was gemfibrozil 1200 mg per day and the mean follow-up was 5.1 years. The concentration of HDL-C was increased by 6% and the plasma triglyceride was decreased by 31% in the gemfibrozil treated group. There was no significant change in concentration of LDL-C.

The primary end point (non-fatal myocardial infarction or death due to CHD) was reduced by 22% from 21.7% in the placebo group to 17.3% in the gemfibrozil group (p=0.006).

An unexpected finding in the VA-HIT study was a significant reduction in stroke in the group treated with gemfibrozil. There were 134 confirmed strokes, 90% of which were ischaemic. Seventy-six occurred in the placebo group (9 fatal) and 58 in the gemfibrozil group (3 fatal), a relative risk reduction of 31%.

The Bezafibrate Infarction Prevention (BIP) study was a five-year, double-blind, placebo-controlled trial that included 3090 subjects with CHD (2825 men, 265 women) aged < 74 years. The concentration of plasma total cholesterol ranged from 182-252 mg/dL (4.7-6.5 mmol/L), the plasma triglyceride concentration was < 300 mg/dL (3.4 mmol/L) and the concentration of HDL-C was < 45 mg/dL (1.16 mmol/L). The active treatment was bezafibrate 400 mg per day. Overall, the study was negative, with no significant effect of bezafibrate on the combined incidence of non-fatal myocardial infarction or death from CHD in the total population. There was, however, a statistically significant reduction in a subgroup of patients whose plasma triglyceride was elevated at entry.

In the subset of patients in whom the concentration of plasma triglyceride at entry into the study was > 200 mg/dL (2.25 mmol/L), the event rate was reduced by 39% from 19.7% in the placebo group to 12.0% in the bezafibrate group (p=0.02).

The Fenofibrate Intervention and Event Lowering in Diabetes (FIELD) study was a five-year, double-blind, placebo controlled clinical trial involving 9,795 patients with type 2 diabetes. The active treatment was micronised fenofibrate given at a dose of 200 mg per day. The baseline lipid levels were total cholesterol 5.04 mmol/L, HDL-C 1.10 mmol/L, TG 1.73 mmol/L and LDL-C 3.07 mmol/L.

Several of the results of the FIELD study were unexpected and remain unexplained. First, the effect of fenofibrate on HDL-C levels was much less than predicted, with the difference between the active and placebo groups being less than 2% at the end of the study. This may have been one of the reasons for the absence of a significant reduction in the primary endpoint of the study (the combined incidence of non-fatal heart attack or death from a coronary event). There were, however, positive outcomes with regard to some of the secondary endpoints. For example, there was an 11% reduction in total cardiovascular events from 13.9% to 12.5% (p=0.035) and a 21% reduction in coronary revascularisation from

7.1% to 5.9% (p=0.003). Stroke, on the other hand, was not significantly reduced by fenofibrate. Nor was there a significant effect on mortality, with 6.6% of the placebo group dying vs 7.3% of the fenofibrate group.

A substantial number of the participants in the FIELD study were commenced on therapy with statins during the trial. Since the uptake of statins was greater in the placebo group (average 17%) than in the fenofibrate group (average 8%), it is likely that the benefits of fenofibrate were masked to some extent by differential statin use between treatment groups.

There were some unpredicted benefits of therapy with fenofibrate in the FIELD study. Patients allocated fenofibrate had less progression of albuminuria (p<0.002). There was also a significantly lower rate of laser treatment for retinopathy (5.2% versus 3.6%, p<0.001), associated with a reduction of macular oedema. This benefit was independent of the presence of prior retinopathy.

The LOpid Coronary Angiography Trial (LOCAT) was a 2.5 year trial that included 395 men who had previously undergone coronary artery bypass surgery. Treatment was slow-release gemfibrozil, 1200 mg once-daily or matching placebo. All subjects underwent baseline coronary angiography, which was repeated after an average of 32 months. Changes in coronary dimensions were assessed by computer-assisted analysis. The change in mean diameter of native coronary segments was -0.04 mm in the placebo group and -0.01 mm in the gemfibrozil group (p=0.009). New lesions in the follow-up angiogram were observed in 23 (14%) of the subjects in the placebo group but in only 4 (2%) of the subjects in the gemfibrozil group (p<0.001).

The Bezafibrate Coronary Atherosclerosis Intervention Trial (BECAIT) was a double-blind, placebo-controlled intervention trial designed to establish whether bezafibrate (200 mg three times daily) could retard or prevent the progression of atherosclerotic lesions in survivors of myocardial infarction. A total of 92 men were randomly assigned to treatment with either bezafibrate or placebo. Coronary angiography was performed at baseline and again after two years and five years.

Bezafibrate changed the concentrations of serum total cholesterol (-9%), VLDL-C (-35%), serum triglyceride (-31%), VLDL triglyceride (-37%) and HDL-C (+9%). The concentration of LDL-C did not change. The mean minimum lumen diameter decreased from baseline to the last angiographic assessment by 0.06 mm in the bezafibrate group and by 0.17 mm in the placebo group, providing a treatment benefit of 0.13 mm (p=0.049). Despite the small number of subjects in the trial, the cumulative coronary event rate was significantly lower in the bezafibrate-treated than in the placebo-treated patients (3 vs 11 patients, respectively; p=0.02).

The Diabetes Atherosclerosis Intervention Study (DAIS) was a three-year angiographic study of 418 men and women with type 2 diabetes who were randomised to receive micronised fenofibrate (200 mg per day) or placebo. The fenofibrate group had a 40% reduction in progression as judged by minimum lumen diameter (p=0.029), 42% less progression as judged by changes in percentage diameter stenosis (p=0.02) and 25% less progression in mean segment diameter (p=0.171, ns).

Trial	Treatment group	Myocardial infarction (fatal plus non-fatal)	Stroke
WHO	Placebo Clofibrate	7.4% 5.9%*	–
HHS	Placebo Gemfibrozil	4.1% 2.7%*	–
VA-HIT	Placebo Gemfibrozil	21.7% 17.3%*	6.9% 5.1%*
BIP	Placebo Bezafibrate	15.0% 13.6%	5.0% 4.6%
FIELD	Placebo Fenofibrate	5.9% 5.2%	3.6% 3.2%

Table XI.2. Cardiovascular outcomes in major fibrate trials

* Statistically significant reduction

Predictors of Benefit in the Fibrate Trials

The cardiovascular benefits of treatment with fibrates appear to be greatest in people with features of the metabolic syndrome.

In the HHS, a baseline level of serum triglyceride > 204 mg/dL (2.3 mmol/L) or an HDL-C < 42 mg/dL (1.08 mmol/L) or a BMI > 26 kg/m^2 identified patients in whom treatment with gemfibrozil produced a reduction in CHD events that was substantially greater than in the study population as a whole. The presence of any one of these factors predicted a 40-50% reduction in CHD events. The presence of all three at baseline identified a group in which there was a massive 78% reduction in CHD events during treatment with gemfibrozil.

As in the HHS, the baseline triglyceride level in the VA-HIT study predicted the magnitude of the CHD reduction achieved by treatment with gemfibrozil. The presence of insulin resistance, with or without diabetes, was also highly predictive of the magnitude of the CHD reduction achieved by treatment with gemfibrozil in VA-HIT.

In the BIP study, with bezafibrate as the active agent, there was no significant reduction in CHD events in the total population. However, in the subset of patients in whom the concentration of plasma triglyceride at entry into the study was > 200 mg/dL (2.25 mmol/L), the event rate was reduced by 39% from 19.7% in the placebo group to 12.0% in the bezafibrate group (p=0.02).

A further post hoc, subgroup analysis of the BIP study found that in 1470 patients with the metabolic syndrome (as defined by ATP-III), bezafibrate was associated with a significant 29% reduction in risk of any myocardial infarction and a significant 33% reduction in non-fatal myocardial infarction. Moreover, in the 575 patients who had four to five components of the metabolic syndrome, bezafibrate was associated with a 56% reduction in the risk of cardiac death (p=0.005).

In line with the HHS, the fenofibrate-mediated reduction in cardiovascular events in the FIELD study was greater in those with lower levels of HDL-C at baseline (< 1.03 mmol/L in men and < 1.29 mmol/L in women) than in those with higher baseline HDL-C levels. Subjects with higher baseline HDL-C levels had a non-significant 4% reduction in total cardiovascular events compared with a significant 14% (p=0.02) reduction in those whose baseline HDL-C levels were lower. The effect of baseline triglyceride levels greater than and less than 200 mg/dL in the FIELD study have not yet been reported.

The subgroup analyses of the HHS, VA-HIT, BIP and FIELD studies suggest that features of the metabolic syndrome (elevated plasma triglyceride, low HDL-C, increased BMI, insulin resistance) identify people in whom fibrates are especially effective in reducing CHD risk.

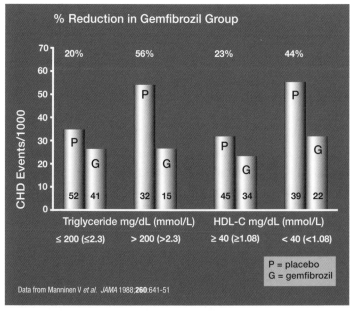

Figure XI.2. Effect of baseline HDL-C and plasma TG on the reduction in CHD events in the Helsinki Heart Study

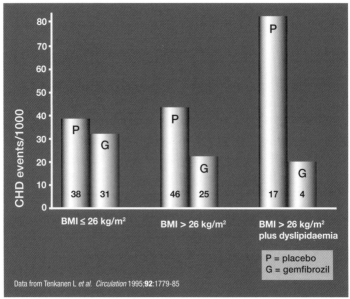

Data from Tenkanen L *et al. Circulation* 1995;**92**:1779-85

Figure XI.3. Effect of baseline BMI in the Helsinki Heart Study

Anti-atherogenic Mechanisms of Fibrates

There are several potential mechanisms by which
fibrates reduce cardiovascular risk. These include
an improvement in dyslipidaemia (reduced plasma
triglyceride, a reduced level of chylomicron and VLDL
remnants, an increase in LDL particle size and an
increase in concentration of HDL-C), an enhancement
of reverse cholesterol transport and direct anti-
inflammatory effects in the artery wall.

Reduced level of plasma triglyceride
Reduced chylomicron and VLDL remnants
Direct anti-inflammatory effects in artery wall
Increased LDL size
Increased reverse cholesterol transport
Increased level of HDL-C

Figure XI.4. Possible anti-atherogenic mechanisms of fibrates

Fibrates increase HDL-C by several mechanisms, all of which are the result of activation of PPARα.
Severe adverse effects of fibrates are rare, although there is a small increase in risk of myositis if a fibrate (especially gemfibrozil) is co-administered with a statin.
Several large-scale clinical trials have demonstrated a reduction in cardiovascular events in people treated with fibrates.
The cardiovascular benefits of treatment with fibrates are greatest in people with features of the metabolic syndrome (low HDL-C, high plasma triglyceride, overweight, insulin resistant).

Table XI.3. Summary

References

Chapman MJ. Fibrates in 2003: therapeutic action in atherogenic dyslipidaemia and future perspectives. *Atherosclerosis* 2003;**171**:1-13.

Barter P. Anti-atherogenic effects of fibrates in type 2 diabetes. *Curr Control Trials Cardiovasc Med* 2001;**2**:218-20.

Rubins HB, Robins SJ, Collins D, Fye CL, Anderson JW, Elam MB, Faas FH, Linares E, Schaefer EJ, Schectman G, Wilt TJ, Wittes J. Gemfibrozil for the secondary prevention of coronary heart disease in men with low levels of high-density lipoprotein cholesterol. Veterans Affairs High-Density Lipoprotein Cholesterol Intervention Trial Study Group. *N Engl J Med* 1999;**341**:410-18.

Rubins HB, Robins SJ, Collins D, Nelson DB, Elam MB, Schaefer EJ, Faas FH, Anderson JW. Diabetes, plasma insulin, and cardiovascular disease: subgroup analysis from the Department of Veterans Affairs high-density lipoprotein intervention trial (VA-HIT). *Arch Intern Med* 2002;**162**:2597-604.

Frick MH, Elo O, Haapa K *et al*. Helsinki Heart Study primary prevention trial with gemfibrozil in middle-aged men with dyslipidemia. *N Engl J Med* 1987;**317**:1237-45.

Tenkanen L, Manttari M, Manninen V. Some coronary risk factors related to the insulin resistance syndrome and treatment with gemfibrozil. Experience from the Helsinki Heart Study. *Circulation* 1995;**92**:1779-85.

Keech A, Simes RJ, Barter P *et al*., on behalf of the field study writing committee. Effects of long-term fenofibrate therapy on cardiovascular events in 9795 people with type 2 diabetes mellitus (the FIELD study): randomised controlled trial. *Lancet* 2005;**366**:1849-61.

The major effect of statins is to reduce the concentration of LDL-C. However, they also have an HDL raising effect, with increases in HDL-C in the order of 5–10% being reported. The dose-response curve for statin-induced increases in HDL-C concentration differs markedly from that of statin-induced LDL-C lowering. Most of the increase in HDL-C is achieved at relatively low doses of statins. In some cases, the effect is already maximal at the lowest recommended dose.

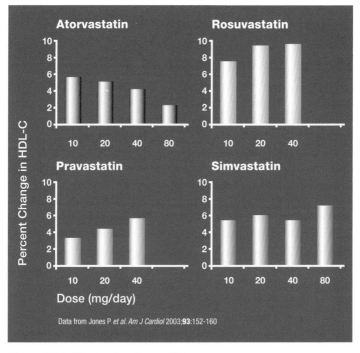

Figure XII.1. Effects of statins on HDLs

Mode of Action of Statins

Statins inhibit 3-hydroxy-3-methylglutaryl coenzyme A (HMG CoA) reductase, the enzyme catalysing the rate-limiting step in cholesterol synthesis. The resulting reduction in cholesterol synthesis stimulates cells to increase their LDL receptor activity and thus enhance their ability to remove LDLs from plasma. This explains why statins lower the level of LDL-C in plasma. However, statins appear also to increase the synthesis of apoA-I by activating PPARα, although the mechanism of activation is indirect and different from that of fibrates. Statins also inhibit CETP, an action that contributes additional HDL raising.

Increased synthesis of apoA-I
Secondary to a reduction in VLDL and LDL
Inhibition of CETP

Table XII.1. Mechanism of HDL-C raising by statins

Variations in the HDL Raising Properties of Different Statins

The increase in HDL-C achieved by statins is generally sustained as the dose of the statin is increased. In the case of atorvastatin, however, the increase in HDL-C falls off at higher doses. The reason for this is not known.

The concentration of HDL-C reflects a balance between processes of synthesis and catabolism of the HDL particles. It is conceivable that the fall-off in concentration of HDL-C at higher doses of atorvastatin is the consequence of an enhanced hepatic uptake of HDL-C rather than a decrease in synthesis of apoA-I. Given that such a hepatic uptake is the final step in the pathway of reverse cholesterol transport and that its stimulation is potentially anti-atherogenic, it is conceivable that the decrease in HDL-C at higher doses of atorvastatin could reflect an enhancement of an anti-atherogenic process. If, however, the fall in HDL-C reflects a decreased synthesis of apoA-I, it may indicate a reduced anti-atherogenic potential. The true situation is currently not known and will have to await further investigation.

Another possible explanation for the observed loss of the HDL raising effect at higher doses of atorvastatin is the fact that major atorvastatin metabolites have potent anti-oxidant properties. It is known that anti-oxidants, such as probucol, reduce HDL-C levels and a mixture of vitamins C and E, beta carotene and selenium has been reported to reduce the HDL raising effects achieved by the combination of simvastatin and niacin. It has also been reported that the ability of statins to raise the level of HDL-C is markedly influenced by paraoxonase genotype of the subject. However, further research is required before concluding that anti-oxidant properties of atorvastatin metabolites contribute to the loss of HDL-C raising when the drug is given at high doses.

Adverse Effects of Statins

Statins are generally extremely well tolerated. The best-known of the adverse effects is myositis, with a reported incidence of about 0.5%. Usually, it is mild and leads to stopping therapy in < 0.1% of cases.

The risk of myositis is increased by simultaneous therapy with cyclosporine, fibrates, macrolide antibiotics, such as erythromycin and conazole anti-fungal agents. The risk is also greater in the elderly, in those with multiple diseases, in the post-operative state and in hypothyroidism. However, there is a consensus that serum creatine kinase (CK) need not be determined routinely. The test is indicated if the patient has unexplained myalgia or muscular symptoms. Concentrations of CK $\geq$ 10 times above the upper limit of the reference value are regarded as significant and, unless otherwise explained, are an indication to suspend therapy. Rechallenge can be considered after the CK has returned to normal.

Liver enzyme levels are increased in about 2% of patients on statins. Most likely, this reflects differences in the metabolism of the enzyme rather than liver damage.

Myositis reported in 0.5%; usually mild, leading to stopping therapy in < 0.1% of cases.
Risk of myositis is increased by simultaneous therapy with cyclosporine, fibrates, macrolide antibiotics such as erythromycin and conazole anti-fungal agents.
Risk of myositis greater in the elderly, in those with multiple diseases, in the post-operative state and in hypothyroidism.
Liver enzyme levels are increased in about 2% of patients on statins. Most likely, this reflects changes in metabolism of the enzyme rather than liver damage.

Table XII.2. Adverse effects of statins

Statin Trials

There are many published primary and secondary prevention studies with statins. Highly positive results have been obtained with simvastatin, pravastatin, lovastatin and atorvastatin. These studies have been conducted in a wide range of patient groups and there is no evidence of any specific group that does not derive benefit from treatment with a statin. In terms of the coronary event reduction achieved with statins, the evidence is clear that most of the benefits are secondary to the reduction in concentration of LDL-C. Any additional risk reduction achieved by the modest statin-induced increase in HDL-C should be viewed as a bonus rather than a major benefit. However, the 8% increase in HDL-C achieved by treatment with simvastatin in the Scandinavian Simvastatin Survival Study (4S) was independently predictive of cardiovascular benefit.

Impact of Statin-induced HDL Raising on CHD

Overall, the relationship between changes in HDL-C and CHD events in the statin end point trials is unclear, probably because it is obscured by the major reduction in LDL-C. If a statin-induced elevation of HDL-C does reduce events, the magnitude of the benefit may be small relative to the protection resulting from the reduction in LDL-C. It is also apparent that such treatment does not eliminate the risk associated with a low HDL, as evidenced by the observations that a low baseline level of HDL-C remains predictive of coronary events in patients treated with statins.

Trial (drug)	Percent reduction in CHD events	Relationship of CHD events to increase in HDL-C	Baseline HDL-C predicts events	
			On placebo	On statin
WOSCOPS (pravastatin)	31	Not significant	yes	yes
AFCAPS/ TexCAPS (lovastatin)	25	Not significant	yes	no
4S (simvastatin)	34	p<0.05	yes	yes
CARE (pravastatin)	24	Not significant	yes	yes
LIPID (pravastatin)	24	Not significant	yes	yes

Table XII.3. Relationship between CHD events and HDL-C in selected statin trials

WOSCOPS - West Of Scotland Coronary Prevention Study

AFCAPS/TexCAPS - Air Force/Texas Coronary Atherosclerosis Prevention Study

4S - Scandinavian Simvastatin Survival Study

CARE - Cholesterol And Recurrent Events trial

LIPID - Long-Term Intervention with Pravastatin in Ischaemic Disease study

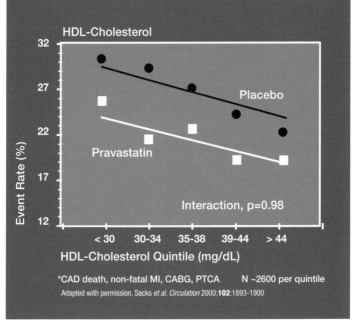

Figure XII.2. Baseline HDL-C and CV events* in placebo and treated groups in the combined LIPID-CARE studies

The relationship between HDL-C raising with statins and the progression/regression of coronary atheroma has been investigated in an analysis of data from 1455 patients in four intravascular ultrasound imaging trials. Statin treatment led to mean LDL-C levels during treatment of 2.3 mmol/L, representing a 23.5% decrease from baseline levels. In addition, statin treatment increased HDL-C by a mean of 7.5%. Changes in HDL-C during treatment were inversely correlated with atheroma progression. Multivariate analysis showed that mean levels of LDL-C and the increase in HDL-C during statin treatment were significant independent predictors of atheroma progression.

The major effect of statins is to reduce the concentration of LDL-C.
The statin-induced reduction in LDL-C accounts for most of the reduction in cardiovascular risk.
Statins also raise HDL-C by 5–10% which also contributes to a reduction in cardiovascular risk.
The main serious adverse effect of statins is myositis but this is rare.
The risk of myositis is increased if co-administered with fibrates (especially gemfibrozil).
While statins decrease cardiovascular risk in all people, regardless of whether the HDL-C is high or low, they do not eliminate the risk associated with a low baseline level of HDL-C.

Table XII.4. Summary

References

Barter PJ. Effects of statins on HDL and the implications for CHD prevention. In: *Lipids and Atherosclerosis Annual 2003,* Martin Dunitz, London, 2003:71-88.

Nicholls SJ, Tuzcu EM, Sipahi I *et al*. Statins, high-density lipoprotein cholesterol, and regression of coronary atherosclerosis. *JAMA* 2007;**297**:499-508.

Niacin (nicotinic acid) has long been used as a lipid-modifying agent. It lowers plasma triglyceride by 40–50%. It lowers LDL-C by up to 20% and increases HDL-C by up to 30%. In terms of its effects on plasma lipids, niacin can be termed a broad-spectrum lipid-modifying agent. However, until recently its widespread therapeutic use has been limited by unpleasant side effects experienced by some people.

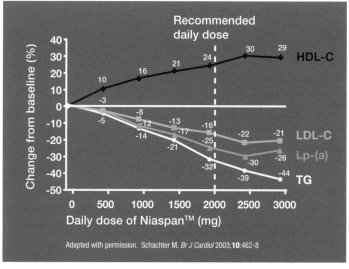

Adapted with permission. Schachter M. *Br J Cardiol* 2003;**10**:462-8

Figure XIII.1. Effects of niacin on HDLs

Mode of HDL Raising Action of Niacin
The precise mechanism of the HDL raising effects of niacin is not known. There is some evidence that part of the effect is secondary to the ability of niacin to lower plasma triglyceride levels and thus reduce the transfer of cholesterol from HDLs to triglyceride-rich lipoproteins. However, this explains only part of the effect. Clearly, the mechanism of the HDL-raising effects of niacin is an important area for further research.

Adverse Effects of Niacin
Most of the adverse effects relate to the use of earlier formulations of niacin that had to be taken in large amounts, divided into three doses each day, with unpleasant episodes of flushing and itching occurring in more than 80% of patients. Dizziness, tachycardia, palpitations and shortness of breath were also common.

New Formulations of Niacin

To a large extent, the flushing problems associated with the original immediate-release forms of niacin have been overcome by the development of newer extended-release niacin formulations such as Niaspan. The extended-release formulations are associated with both a lower incidence and severity of the unpleasant effects of the original forms.

While flushing and itching still occur in a proportion of patients taking extended-release niacin, the frequency is much less and the problem is often transient, disappearing with continued use. The reason for the improved tolerance of extended-release niacin relates, in part, to the lower dose required to achieve equivalent lipid modifications but also relates to the rate at which the agent is delivered to the liver. The frequency and severity of flushing with extended-release forms of niacin can be further reduced by initiating therapy with low doses and slowly titrate to a full therapeutic dose over several weeks. Hepatic problems encountered with an earlier, much more sustained-release form of the niacin, have not been observed with extended-release niacin such as Niaspan.

Another more slowly absorbed coated formulation of extended-release niacin (Niaspan) is associated with an even greater reduction in flushing than with previous formulations.

Aspirin taken 30 minutes before taking niacin further reduces niacin-induced flushing.

Combination of Extended Release Niacin with Laropiprant

An additional novel approach to reducing the flushing associated with niacin is currently under investigation. This involves the co-administration of an extended-release formulation of niacin with a new drug named laropiprant. Laropiprant is a selective antagonist of the prostaglandin D(2) receptor subtype 1 (DP_1) that is thought to mediate niacin-induced vasodilation. By inhibiting the DP_1 receptor, laropiprant suppresses both subjective and objective manifestations of niacin-induced vasodilation. The cardioprotective properties of the combination of extended-release niacin plus laropiprant are currently being tested in a very large clinical trial named HPS2-THRIVE (see pages 75–76 for details).

Use of Niacin in Diabetes and Insulin Resistant States

Reports that niacin may reduce insulin sensitivity and thus be contraindicated in insulin resistant states such as type 2 diabetes and the metabolic syndrome have not turned out to be a significant problem. There is no reason in clinical practice to withhold Niaspan from subjects with diabetes or insulin resistance.

Flushing
Dizziness
Tachycardia
Palpitations

Table XIII.1. Adverse effects of niacin

Clinical Relevance of HDL-C Raising by Niacin

Early studies: Two early clinical trials demonstrated a benefit of niacin in the prevention of cardiovascular disease. The Coronary Drug Project (CDP) involved the treatment of patients with myocardial infarction with a daily dose of 3 g niacin for a total of 6.5 years. Major CHD events were significantly reduced by 14%. While there was no significant reduction in mortality at the end of the trial, in an analysis of the 15-year follow-up data there was a statistically significant reduction in total mortality in the group originally allocated to the niacin group. The relationship of benefit to the HDL raising achieved with niacin in this study was not reported.

Another early study was the Stockholm Ischaemic Heart Disease Secondary Prevention Study in which survivors of myocardial infarction were randomised at discharge from hospital into one of two groups: one was an untreated control group and the other received 3 g per day niacin and 2 g per day clofibrate. The study lasted five years. The combined treatment with niacin and clofibrate was accompanied by a statistically significant reduction in both total (26% reduction) and CHD (36% reduction) mortality. Again, however, the relationship of the benefit to any HDL raising was not reported.

Two more recent studies have focused more on the HDL raising effects of niacin. In each of these, a niacin-induced increase in HDL-C, especially if co-administered with a statin, was associated with a reduction in both coronary atherosclerosis and coronary events.

The HDL Atherosclerosis Treatment Study (HATS) was a double-blind, three-year angiographic study investigating the effects of simvastatin plus niacin in 160 patients with coronary disease and low plasma levels of HDL. Treatment with the combination of simvastatin and niacin reduced LDL-C by 42% and increased HDL-C by 26%. The average coronary stenosis progressed by 3.9% with placebo and regressed by 0.4% with simvastatin-niacin (p<0.001). The frequency of a clinical cardiovascular end point was 24% in the placebo group and 3% with simvastatin-niacin. Despite the small number of subjects in the trial, this difference was statistically highly significant.

ARterial Biology for the Investigation of the Treatment Effects of Reducing cholesterol (ARBITER) 2 is a recent study showing cardioprotective benefits of niacin (once-daily extended-release form given in patients also receiving a statin) beyond that achieved with statin monotherapy. ARBITER 2 was a double-blind, randomised, placebo-controlled study in which a once-daily 1000 mg dose of extended-release niacin (Niaspan) was added to background statin therapy in 167 patients with known CHD and low levels of HDL-C (< 45 mg/dL). The primary end point was the change in common carotid intima-media thickness (CIMT) after one year. Adherence to Niaspan was excellent with 149 subjects completing the study. The level of HDL-C increased by 21% in the Niaspan-treated group. After 12 months, mean CIMT increased significantly by 0.044 mm in the placebo group but was unchanged in the niacin group. The overall difference in CIMT progression between the Niaspan and placebo groups approached statistical significance (p=0.08). In the group of subjects without insulin resistance, the positive effects of Niaspan did reach statistical significance (p=0.026).

The results of ARBITER 2 have been extended in ARBITER 3, a 12-month follow-up of 130 of the subjects who had participated in ARBITER 2. During this follow-up, all subjects received the combination of a statin plus Niaspan at a dose of 1000 mg per day. This therapy resulted in a significant decrease in CIMT compared with baseline (-0.04 ± 0.014 mm; p=0.008).

It is apparent that niacin is an extremely effective HDL raising agent that, especially when co-administered with a statin, results not only in favourable lipid changes but also in a substantial reduction in atherosclerosis and cardiovascular events. This proposition is being put to the test in a major new clinical trial.

Ongoing Clinical Trials with Niacin
The Atherothrombosis Intervention in Metabolic Syndrome with Low HDL-C/High Triglyceride and Impact on Global Health Outcomes (AIM-HIGH) study has commenced and will include 3300 people with established vascular disease and dyslipidaemia (low HDL-C and high triglyceride). AIM-HIGH is a six-year study designed to determine whether the combination of an extended-release form of niacin (Niaspan) and simvastatin is superior to simvastatin alone in preventing cardiovascular events. This study will provide important information about the benefits of simultaneously raising HDL-C and lowering LDL-C. The results of this trial should be available in about 2012.

Treatment of HDL to Reduce the Incidence of Vascular Events (HPS2-THRIVE) is a very large trial involving 20000 people with established cardiovascular disease and who are therefore at very high risk of having a further cardiovascular event. It has already commenced and will be completed in 2013. All participants will receive effective LDL-lowering therapy (either simvastatin 40 mg daily alone or with ezetimibe 10 mg daily in a combination tablet). Eligible subjects will then be randomised to receive either a placebo or the combination of extended-release niacin plus laropiprant. This trial is planned to complete in 2013 and will reveal whether raising HDL-C with niacin translates into a reduction in the risk of having a cardiovascular event over and above that achieved by highly effective LDL-C lowering therapy.

An Assessment of Coronary Health using an Intima-media thickness Endpoint for Vascular Effects (ACHIEVE) is a two-year multinational study designed to assess the effect of the combination of extended-release niacin plus laropiprant on changes in carotid artery intima-media thickness as assessed by B-mode ultrasound. Nine hundred patients with heterozygous familial hypercholesterolaemia will be enrolled in the study. All will be on effective LDL-C lowering therapy before being randomised in a double-blind fashion to receive either the combination of extended-release niacin plus laropiprant or matching placebo for up to 96 weeks. Patients are currently being screened for inclusion in this study.

Conclusions

> Although statin therapy is effective in lowering LDL-C, residual CVD risk remains after statin therapy.

> Lipid abnormalities beyond LDL-C (non–HDL-C, TG, HDL-C) should be intensively treated to reduce residual CVD risk.

> Clinical trial data support the efficacy of niacin for reducing CVD risk when used alone and in combination with statins.

> Niacin/statin combination therapy corrects all atherogenic lipid abnormalities and slows the progression and increases the regression of coronary atherosclerosis.

> Niacin has been in clinical use for four decades with an established safety profile, including its use in combination therapy with statins.

Niacin (nicotinic acid) increases HDL-C by up to 30%, lowers plasma triglyceride by 40-50% and lowers LDL-C by up to 20%.
Niacin increases the synthesis of both apoA-I and apoA-II.
Adverse effects of niacin include flushing, dizziness, tachycardia and palpitations.
These adverse effects are reduced with Niaspan, a prolonged-release form of the drug.
Clinical trials with niacin have been associated with a reduction in cardiovascular events and with a reduction in progression of atherosclerosis.

Table XIII.2. Summary

References

Carlson LA. Niaspan, the prolonged release preparation of nicotinic acid (niacin), the broad-spectrum lipid drug. *Int J Clin Pract* 2004;**58**:706-13.

McGovern ME. Use of nicotinic acid in patients with elevated fasting glucose, diabetes, or metabolic syndrome. *Br J Diabetes Vasc Dis* 2004;**4**:78-83.

Chapman MJ, Assmann G, Fruchart JC, Shepherd J, Sirtori C; European Consensus Panel on HDL-C. Raising high-density lipoprotein cholesterol with reduction of cardiovascular risk: the role of nicotinic acid — a position paper developed by the European Consensus Panel on HDL-C. *Curr Med Res Opin* 2004;**20**:1253-68.

Brown BG, Zhao XQ, Chait A *et al*. Simvastatin and niacin, anti-oxidant vitamins, or the combination for the prevention of coronary disease. *N Engl J Med* 2001;**345**:1583-92.

Taylor AJ, Sullenberger LE, Lee HJ, Lee JK, Grace KA. Arterial biology for the investigation of the treatment effects of reducing cholesterol (ARBITER) 2. A double-blind, placebo controlled study of extended-release niacin on atherosclerosis progression in secondary prevention patients treated with statins. *Circulation* 2004;**110**:3512-17.

McKenney J. New perspectives on the use of niacin in the treatment of lipid disorders. *Arch Intern Med* 2004;**164**:697-705.

Cefali EA, Simmons PD, Stanek EJ, Shamp TR. Improved control of niacin-induced flushing using an optimized once-daily, extended-release niacin formulation. *Int J Clin Pharmacol Ther* 2006;**44**:633-40.

CETP promotes the transfer of cholesterol from the protective HDL fraction to potentially pro-atherogenic particles in the VLDL/LDL fractions. Its inhibition results in an increase in the concentration of HDL-C and a decrease in VLDL-C and LDL-C.

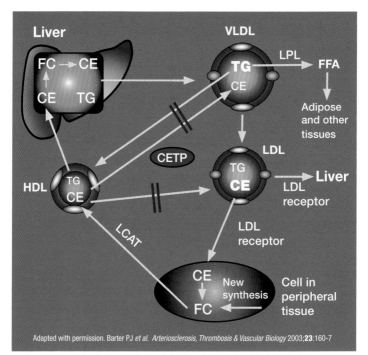

Adapted with permission. Barter PJ *et al. Arteriosclerosis, Thrombosis & Vascular Biology* 2003;**23**:160-7

Figure XIV.1. Effect of inhibiting CETP on plasma cholesterol transport

CETP inhibition increases concentration of HDL-C resulting in an:
• increase in the efflux of cholesterol from plaques
• enhancement of the anti-inflammatory effects of HDL
• enhancement of the anti-oxidant effects of HDL

CETP inhibition decreases concentration of LDL cholesterol

CETP inhibition decreases the cholesterol content of triglyceride-rich lipoproteins, rendering them less atherogenic

Figure XIV.2. Anti-atherogenic effects of inhibiting CETP: potential mechanisms

CETP inhibition has been shown in several studies to be markedly anti-atherogenic in rabbits.

Rabbits have high level of activity of CETP
Rabbits naturally highly susceptible to the development of atherosclerosis
Inhibition of CETP in rabbits decreases atherosclerosis

Figure XIV.3. Effects of inhibiting CETP on development of atherosclerosis in rabbits

Drugs that inhibit CETP have been developed and tested in humans. One of these, torcetrapib, increased HDL-C by more than 50% and decreased LDL-C by about 20%. A consistent finding in the torcetrapib studies has been a small but significant increase in systolic and diastolic blood pressure by a still unknown mechanism.

The magnitude of the increase in HDL-C in people treated with torcetrapib, combined with the observed vascular benefits of CETP inhibition in rabbits, led to decisions to conduct major clinical trials with torcetrapib. Specifically, these trials were designed to test whether inhibiting CETP in humans translated into a reduction in cardiovascular risk over and above that achieved with effective treatment with statins.

The largest of these studies was the **Investigation of Lipid Level management to Understand its iMpact IN ATherosclerotic Events (ILLUMINATE)** trial that was designed to investigate possible cardioprotective effects of inhibiting CETP with torcetrapib. This trial had to be terminated early because of an excess of deaths in the torcetrapib-treated group.

The ILLUMINATE trial included 15000 people with manifest cardiovascular disease or type-2 diabetes. All were treated with atorvastatin at a dose necessary to reduce the LDL-C level to less than 100 mg/dL (2.6 mmol/L) before being randomised in a double-blind fashion to receive torcetrapib 60 mg per day or matching placebo. The follow-up was estimated to be 4.5 years in order to achieve enough events to test the hypothesis that treatment with torcetrapib was cardioprotective. This trial was terminated in December 2006 after a median follow-up of only 18 months because of an excess of deaths in the group treated with torcetrapib. The number of deaths was 82 in the torcetrapib arm, compared to 51 deaths in the control arm. This difference was statistically significant. The explanation for the excess mortality is currently not known.

Question: What do the safety issues in ILLUMINATE mean for the HDL hypothesis?

Answer: There is nothing in the ILLUMINATE trial to invalidate the HDL hypothesis.

Three imaging trials had just been completed at around the time the ILLUMINATE trial was terminated. In all three studies, patients had been treated with atorvastatin to achieve optimal levels of LDL-C before being randomised to receive torcetrapib at a daily-dose of 60 mg or matching placebo. All subjects continued on atorvastatin throughout the trial. The treatments were continued for two years.

One of these trials, **Investigation of Lipid Level Management Using Coronary Ultrasound to Assess Reduction of Atherosclerosis by CETP Inhibition and HDL Elevation (ILLUSTRATE)** involved the use of intravascular ultrasound to assess the effect of torcetrapib on coronary atheroma burden while the other two, **Rating Atherosclerotic Disease Change by Imaging with A New CETP Inhibitor (RADIANCE) 1** and **2**, used ultrasound to assess the effects of torcetrapib on carotid intima-media thickness. The ILLUSTRATE trial involved people with demonstrable coronary atheroma, while RADIANCE 1 and 2 trials involved patients with familial hypercholesterolaemia and mixed hyperlipidaemia, respectively.

The results of all three trials were essentially the same, with no evidence that addition of torcetrapib to atorvastatin provided any benefits over and above those of atorvastatin alone. But, nor was there any evidence of harm.

So, what can be learnt from the imaging trials?

The imaging trials certainly indicate that torcetrapib does not promote regression of atherosclerosis in either coronary or carotid arteries. But the fact that they showed no evidence of progression of disease means that they provided no evidence of harm and thus cannot help in understanding the cause of the excess of deaths in the torcetrapib arm in the ILLUMINATE trial.

Question: Does CETP inhibition have a therapeutic future after torcetrapib?

The crucial question is: were the excess deaths in the torcetrapib arm of the ILLUMINATE trial due to CETP inhibition or were they the result of an unknown serious adverse effect of torcetrapib unrelated to CETP inhibition? If the former, there is clearly no future for CETP inhibition as a therapeutic strategy. If, however, the problem was an off-target effect of torcetrapib that is not shared with other CETP inhibitors, then the class retains its potential, even if the task of proving therapeutic benefit is made more difficult.

So, what should we do?

We know that there exists an unacceptably high residual risk of cardiovascular events in some people despite aggressive statin therapy and that this risk is partly attributable to low HDL levels. So, the case for HDL-raising therapy is compelling.

But is CETP inhibition the right way to proceed?

The answer to this will depend on resolution of the following issues.

1. It is essential to investigate possible off-target adverse effects of torcetrapib, including the basis of the increase in blood pressure in people taking the drug. Clues may be provided after the ILLUMINATE trial results have been fully analysed. Such clues may then direct further basic research into understanding the mechanism underlying the adverse effects.

2. If an off-target adverse effect of torcetrapib can be established and its mechanism understood, it will be necessary to show beyond reasonable doubt that other CETP inhibitors do not share this adverse effect.

3. If the problem with torcetrapib was an off-target effect of known mechanism and if other CETP inhibitors can be shown not to have such an effect, then there is a compelling case for continuing to pursue CETP as an anti-atherogenic strategy by conducting both imaging and large-scale outcome trials.

References

Barter PJ, Brewer HB Jr, Chapman MJ, Hennekens CH, Rader DJ, Tall AR. Cholesteryl ester transfer protein: a novel target for raising HDL and inhibiting atherosclerosis. *Arterioscler Thromb Vasc Biol* 2003;**23**:160-7.

Nissen SE, Tardif JC, Nicholls SJ *et al.*: ILLUSTRATE Investigators. Effect of torcetrapib on the progression of coronary atherosclerosis. *N Engl J Med* 2007;**356**:1304-16.

Kastelein JJ, van Leuven SI, Burgess L *et al.*: RADIANCE 1 Investigators. Effect of torcetrapib on carotid atherosclerosis in familial hypercholesterolaemia. *N Engl J Med* 2007;**356**:1620-30.

Bots ML, Visseren FL, Evans GW *et al.* Torcetrapib and carotid intima-media thickness in mixed dyslipidaemia (RADIANCE 2 study): a randomised, double-blind trial. *Lancet* 2007;**370**:153-60.

15 Selective Cannabinoid Type 1 Receptor Blockers

Selective cannabinoid type 1 (CB_1) receptor blockers are agents that have the ability to correct the multiple cardiometabolic risk factors that are present in many overweight or obese people. They may also help promote smoking cessation. CB_1 receptors are components of the recently discovered endocannabinoid system. They play an important role in food intake, energy balance and are directly implicated in lipid and glucose metabolism. Overactivity of the endocannabinoid system may lead to the development of abdominal obesity and its associated cardiovascular risk factors, including atherogenic dyslipidaemia, insulin resistance and type 2 diabetes, high blood pressure and a pro-inflammatory state.

Early experience in clinical trials with the first selective CB_1 receptor blocker (rimonabant) has been most encouraging. Blockade of CB_1 receptor centrally (in brain) and peripherally (in adipocytes, liver, muscle and gastro-intestinal tract) leads to a reduction in body weight and waist circumference, an elevation of HDL-C, a reduction of plasma triglyceride and an improvement in insulin sensitivity. These effects have been shown in large clinical trials to be sustained for up to two years. Indeed, HDL-C increases of up to 25% have been observed in people treated with rimonabant, an effect substantially greater than that predicted from the associated weight loss.

Rimonabant is a promising new agent that has the potential to improve multiple cardiometabolic risk factors, including low HDL-C, in people with abdominal obesity.

References

Henness S, Robinson DM, Lyseng-Williamson KA. Rimonabant. *Drugs* 2006;**66**:2109-19.

Despres JP, Golay A, Sjostrom L; Rimonabant in Obesity-Lipids Study Group. Effects of rimonabant on metabolic risk factors in overweight patients with dyslipidemia. *N Engl J Med* 2005;**353**:2121-34.

How is Low HDL-C Defined?

The population studies indicate that the higher the level of HDL-C, the lower the risk of having a cardiovascular event. There is no single concentration of HDL-C that defines a sudden change in risk. Thus, any definition of low HDL-C is arbitrary. Many guidelines suggest that an HDL-C < 40 mg/dL (1.03 mmol/L) in men and < 45 mg/dL (1.16 mmol/L) in women should be regarded as low and thus, possibly, warrant HDL raising therapy.

It is possible, however, that the higher the level of HDL-C the better and that high risk people with HDL levels above those recommended in guidelines may still derive benefits from having their level of HDL-C increased further. More research will be required before being able to state with confidence what should be the optimum level of HDL-C.

When should a Low HDL-C be Treated?

As with LDL-C lowering therapy, a decision to use drug therapy in someone with a low HDL-C should be based on the global risk and not solely on the level of HDL-C.

How should a Low HDL-C be Treated?

Lifestyle measures should be recommended in all people with low levels of HDL-C and should include dietary modification, increased physical activity, weight reduction if overweight and smoking cessation if a smoker.

However, all too often, lifestyle changes are not adopted and, even if they are, are not sustained. Furthermore, in many people the HDL-C level remains low despite adoption of appropriate lifestyle measures. Under these circumstances, pharmacological approaches must be considered. The question then is: which drug?

Who should Receive a Fibrate?

The low HDL-C person likely to get the greatest benefit from therapy with a fibrate is someone in whom a high CHD risk is secondary to the presence of type 2 diabetes or features of the metabolic syndrome such as an elevated level of plasma triglyceride. While fibrate-induced increases in HDL-C in such people may be modest, the resulting reduction in CHD events (at least with gemfibrozil) tends to be substantially greater than predicted from the lipid changes.

Who should Receive a Statin?
There is an overwhelming body of evidence from controlled, randomised, clinical trials to indicate that cardiovascular risk is reduced by statin therapy in everyone who takes the medication. However, the evidence also supports a view that the major proportion of this benefit derives from the reduction in LDL-C. While a statin-induced increase in HDL-C will most likely add to the protection, statins do not eliminate the increased risk associated with a low baseline level of HDL-C. Thus, statins should be used primarily as LDL lowering agents with any increase in HDL-C being regarded as a bonus.

Who should Receive Niacin?
Niacin is the most effective, currently available HDL-C raising agent and should be considered in all high risk subjects in whom the level of HDL-C is low.

Should Combinations of Lipid-modifying Drugs be Considered?
Given that the use of lipid-modifying drugs should be limited to people whose risk of CHD is high and given that treatment with statins has been shown to reduce such risk regardless of lipid levels, it follows that all high risk people should be given statins. However, in many people, statins do not correct a low level of HDL-C. Furthermore, statins do not remove the excess risk associated with a low baseline HDL-C, especially in those with features of the metabolic syndrome.

Thus, in high risk people with a low HDL-C, especially when present as a component of insulin resistant states such as the metabolic syndrome or type 2 diabetes, there is a strong case for adding a fibrate to the statin therapy. This case is currently being tested in a trial named Action to Control Cardiovascular Risk in Diabetes (ACCORD) that is investigating whether the combination of fenofibrate plus simvastatin is superior to simvastatin alone to reduce cardiovascular events in people with diabetes.

In the light of the results of the ARBITER 2 study, Niaspan should also be seriously considered as a supplement to statin therapy in those whose low HDL-C is not corrected by the statin.

Caution with the Combination of Fibrates and Statins
The combination of fibrates and statins is associated with a small but significant increased risk of myositis. This risk is greatest when statins are combined with gemfibrozil but is much less when the fibrate is fenofibrate or bezafibrate.

Most guidelines define low HDL-C as: < 40 mg/dL (1.03 mmol/L) in men < 45 mg/dL (1.16 mmol/L) in women
A decision to initiate HDL-C drug therapy should be based on the global risk and not simply on the HDL-C level.
Lifestyle measures should be recommended in all people with low HDL-C.
Fibrates are recommended in the management of low HDL states when the low HDL is present as a component of type 2 diabetes or the metabolic syndrome.
Statins reduce cardiovascular risk in all patients but most of this benefit is secondary LDL-C lowering rather than HDL-C raising.
Niacin is the most effective of the currently available HDL raising drugs and should be considered in high risk subjects with low HDL-C.
Combination therapy with a statin and fibrate should be considered in high risk people with the metabolic syndrome or type 2 diabetes.
Combination therapy with a fibrate and a statin is associated with a small but significant increase in risk of myositis.
Combination therapy with a statin and niacin (in the form of Niaspan) should be considered in people in whom a low HDL-C is not corrected by the statin monotherapy.

Table XVII.1. Summary

Intravenous infusions of reconstituted HDLs (comprising complexes of apoA-I and phospholipids) have already been shown in human trials to improve endothelial function and to promote regression of coronary artery atheroma. However, one limitation of this approach relates to the logistics of obtaining the very large amounts of apoA-I required to make the reconstituted HDLs.

It may be possible to overcome this problem of supply by developing smaller peptides that mimic the action of apoA-I. Studies of several of these so-called HDL mimetics are currently underway in animal models but nothing is yet reported in humans.

Another approach of great importance involves the development of new selective PPAR-α agonists that have all of the beneficial effects of fibrates without the adverse effects. Such agents are already in early stage trials in humans.

Other potential therapeutic targets for therapies designed to elevate the concentration of apoA-I/HDLs include the liver X receptor (LXR), the ABC transporters and other novel agents that appear to increase the synthesis of apoA-I by different mechanisms.

The potential of these new approaches is considerable and results in humans are awaited with great interest.

Despite the impressive CHD risk reduction that has been achieved by statin-induced reductions in LDL-C, the residual risk remains unacceptably high. There is clearly a need now to move beyond LDL-C and statins. This need will become even more pressing as the epidemic of type 2 diabetes and the metabolic syndrome continues to escalate.

The evidence is now overwhelming that HDL raising should be the new target. We already have tools for raising HDL-C, with even more effective agents likely to become available in the not too distant future.

Thus, the time has come for intervening to raise the level of HDL-C in high risk subjects with the same aggression as is currently applied to lowering LDL-C.